MAYO CLINIC

ON BETTER
HEARING
AND BALANCE

Wayne Olsen, Ph.D.

Medical Editor-in-Chief

Mayo Clinic
Rochester, Minnesota

Published by Mayo Clinic Health Solutions

For bulk sales to employers, member groups and health-related companies, contact Mayo Clinic Health Solutions, 200 First St. SW, Rochester, MN, 55905, or send an e-mail to *SpecialSalesMayoBooks@Mayo.edu*.

Address inquiries to Mayo Clinic Health Solutions, Permissions Department, 200 First St. SW, Fifth Floor Centerplace Building, Rochester, MN, 55905.

Stock photography from BananaStock, Brand X Pictures, Comstock, Corbis, Creatas, Digital Stock, Digital Vision, Image Ideas, © Isabelle Rozenbaum/PhotoAlto, Photodisc, Rubberball and Stockbyte. The individuals pictured are models, and the photos are used for illustrative purposes only. There's no correlation between the individuals portrayed and the conditions or subjects being discussed.

Photos on page 132 courtesy of Paws With A Cause, page 149 courtesy of Cochlear Americas, and pages 189 and 191 courtesy of Ultratec

Library of Congress Control Number: 2008927433

Printed in Canada

First Edition

3 4 5 6 7 8 9 10

About Mayo Clinic

Mayo Clinic evolved from the frontier practice of Dr. William Worrall Mayo and the partnership of his two sons, William J. and Charles H. Mayo, in the early 1900s. Pressed by the demands of their busy practice in Rochester, Minn., the Mayo brothers invited other physicians to join them, pioneering the private group practice of medicine. Today, with more than 2,000 physicians and scientists at three major locations in Rochester, Minn., Jacksonville, Fla., and Phoenix and Scottsdale, Ariz., Mayo Clinic is dedicated to providing comprehensive diagnoses, accurate answers and effective treatments.

With this depth of medical knowledge, experience and expertise, Mayo Clinic occupies an unparalleled position as a health information resource. Since 1983, Mayo Clinic has published reliable health information for millions of consumers through a variety of award-winning newsletters, books and online services. Revenue from these publishing activities supports Mayo Clinic programs, including medical education and medical research.

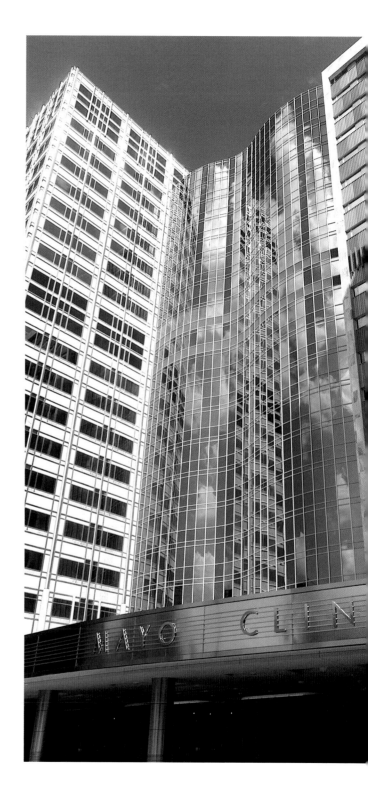

Editorial staff

Preface

Hearing loss and dizziness are two of the most common reasons to visit your doctor. Hearing loss may be present at birth or hereditary. Dizziness may be a solitary symptom or it may be the most debilitating of multiple symptoms. Frequently, hearing loss and balance problems are complications of illness or disease, powerful medication, trauma, noise exposure and the normal process of aging.

This book describes the sensitive structures and exquisite functions of the ear, which is so fundamental to good hearing and balance. Attention is focused on many common ear disorders and the ear-related problems of tinnitus and dizziness. Explanations are provided for diagnostic tests, medical treatment, surgery and rehabilitation. This content helps you become a more informed participant in effective prevention and treatment strategies.

When hearing loss cannot be alleviated medically, many electronic and digital devices are available to help you communicate more easily. Hearing aids, cochlear implants and assistive listening devices are discussed in separate chapters. The treatment and management of balance problems are discussed in the final chapter.

Audiologists and ear, nose and throat specialists at Mayo Clinic facilities in Minnesota, Florida, and Arizona, have reviewed the content of this book for accuracy and completeness. The result is a practical resource to assist you in protecting and preserving your hearing, maintaining your mobility and balance, and minimizing the impact of hearing loss, dizziness and imbalance on your daily life.

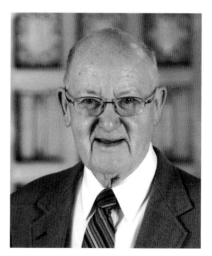

Wayne Olsen, Ph.D.
Medical Editor-in-Chief

Table of contents

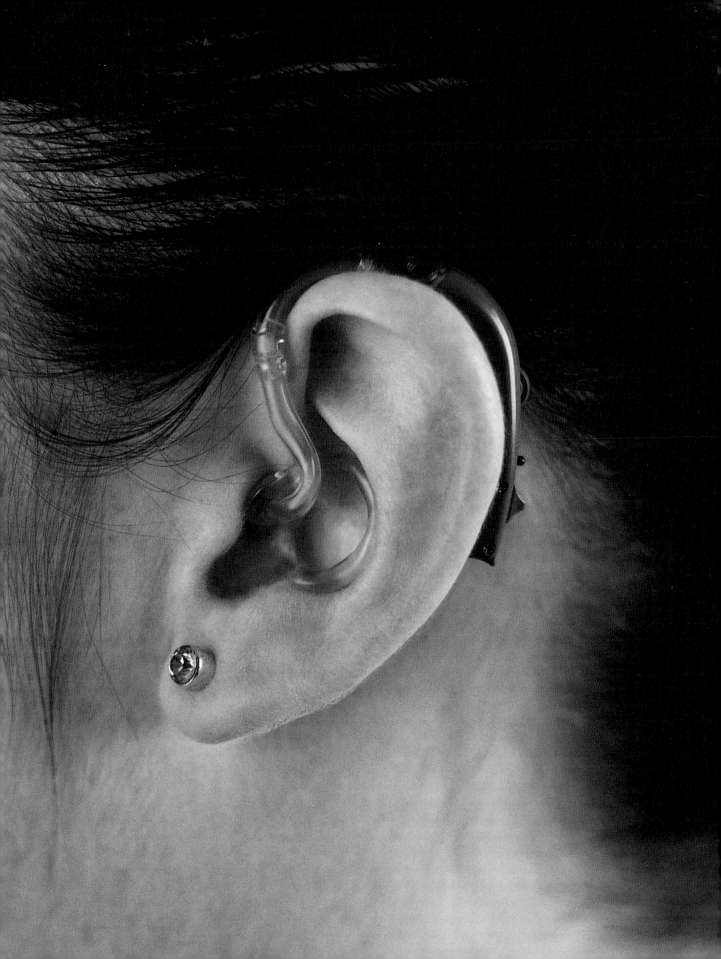

Part 1

Understanding common hearing problems

How you hear

In 1802 the famed German composer Ludwig van Beethoven wrote a letter to his brothers about his deteriorating hearing: "I am compelled to live as an exile. If I approach near to people, a feeling of hot anxiety comes over me lest my condition should be noticed."[1] It's striking that such feelings belonged to a composer whose music, more than two centuries later, still brings so much listening enjoyment to people around the world.

But if you're experiencing problems with hearing, you, like Beethoven, may feel uncomfortable when you're in social situations and conversing with others. Not being able to hear clearly can be frustrating, to say the least, as you try to maintain the conversation.

Hearing loss can cause social isolation because you may find it easier to withdraw from group activities rather than participate in them. Such behavior might in turn cause people to think of you as timid or disconnected and give up trying to communicate with you.

Then again, if you have hearing loss, you have plenty of company. At least 10 percent of Americans — 30 million — have some degree of hearing loss, ranging from mild to profound.

[1] *Eaglefield-Hull, A., ed.* Beethoven's Letters. *New York: Dover Publications; 1972:38.*

Older adults are most affected, as hearing tends to deteriorate with age. An estimated 30 percent of Americans age 65 and older, and approximately 50 percent of those over age 75, have a hearing impairment. But hearing loss can occur at any age due to factors such as noise exposure, trauma, genetics and illness. Worldwide, the number of people with hearing loss is estimated at 500 million.

Many people refuse to acknowledge hearing loss. Estimates are that only about one person in four who would benefit from a hearing aid actually wears one. Many choose to persevere without any assistance.

According to a study from the National Council on Aging, people with hearing impairment who don't use hearing aids are more likely to feel sad or anxious, be less active socially and feel greater emotional insecurity than are those with hearing impairment who do use hearing aids. The study also reported that hearing aid users maintained better relationships with their families.

Hearing aids have come a long way since the conspicuous ear trumpets of the 18th and 19th centuries. In fact, astounding improvements in hearing technology have been made in the last few decades. More options for treating hearing loss are available. And some of these options are not even noticeable to onlookers. The key is to find a treatment that fits your needs and lifestyle.

In the chapters that follow, you'll find pertinent information about hearing loss — why it occurs, how it's diagnosed, how it can be treated and how you can live with it. You'll also learn about dizziness and problems with balance, conditions that sometimes are associated with hearing difficulties. This knowledge will help you live an active life despite any changes that may occur to your hearing.

Structure of the ear

The ears are pretty amazing acoustic devices, as yet unmatched by human ingenuity or invention. In a person with normal hearing, the ears, in combination with the brain, can almost instantly transform sound waves from the external world into the recognizable voice of a loved one, the call of a songbird or a crack of thunder.

Many factors play into this sensory organ, so let's take a systematic look at the important structures that make up the ear. The flap of cartilage on each side of your head may be the most recognizable structure, but that's only the external part of the ear. The organ that you use for hearing is actually composed of three complex, interconnected sections known as the outer ear, middle ear and inner ear.

Outer ear

The outer ear is the part of the organ you can see sticking out from either side of your head. It's made up of folds of skin and cartilage, called the pinna (auricle), and the ear canal. The cupped shape of the pinna (PIN-uh) gathers sound waves from the environment and directs them toward the ear canal.

The ear canal is an inch-long passageway leading to the eardrum. The skin lining the ear canal contains tiny hairs and glands that produce wax, or cerumen (suh-ROO-mun). The hairs and wax serve as cleaning mechanisms for the ear canal by repelling water, protecting against bacteria and keeping foreign objects such as dirt from slipping through the ear canal and reaching the eardrum.

The eardrum (tympanic membrane) is a thin, taut membrane at the end of the ear canal that separates the outer ear from the middle ear. The arrival of sound waves through the ear canal will cause the eardrum to vibrate.

Middle ear

The middle ear is an air-filled cavity located behind the eardrum. The cavity is lodged in the temporal bone of your skull and houses three tiny bones called ossicles (OS-ih-kuls). The ossicles have scientific names, but each is known by a name that best describes its shape: the hammer (malleus), anvil (incus) and stirrup (stapes). See the illustration on page 16.

Together, the ossicles form a bridge between the eardrum and the membrane-covered entrance to the inner ear (oval window). Sound waves are transmitted through the ossicles. Each bone moves back and forth, much as a small lever, to increase the sound level that reaches the inner ear. A tiny muscle is attached to the hammer on one end of the ossicular bridge, and another tiny muscle to the stirrup at the other end.

A narrow channel called the eustachian (u-STA-shun) tube connects the middle

Parts of the ear

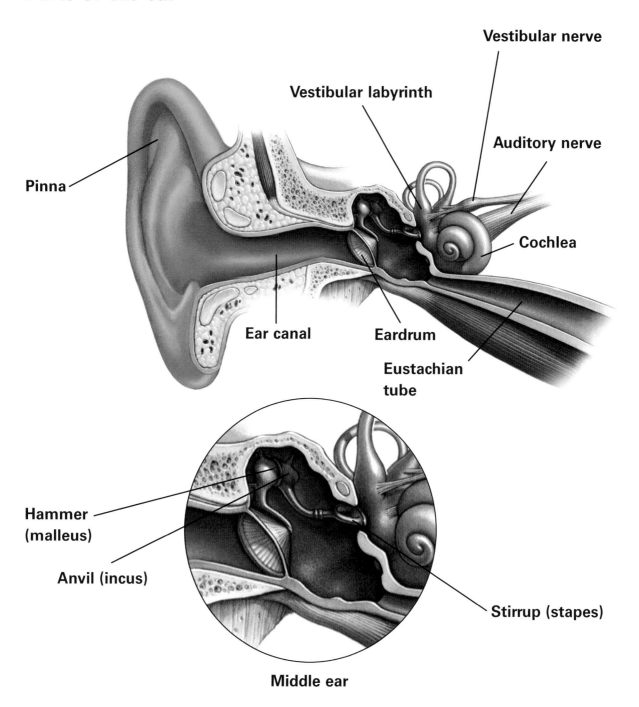

Vestibular nerve

Vestibular labyrinth

Auditory nerve

Pinna

Cochlea

Ear canal

Eardrum

Eustachian tube

Hammer (malleus)

Anvil (incus)

Stirrup (stapes)

Middle ear

ear to back of the nose and upper part of the throat — an area called the nasopharynx (na-zo-FAR-inks).

The eustachian tube normally remains closed until you swallow or yawn. Then it opens briefly to equalize the air pressure within your middle ear to the air pressure that's outside — you may feel and hear a pop when this occurs. Maintaining equal air pressure on both sides of the eardrum allows the membrane to vibrate easily.

In adults, the eustachian tube angles slightly downward to the nasopharynx. In children, because their skulls aren't yet fully developed, the eustachian tube is narrower and more horizontal. This makes it easier for a child's eustachian tube to become blocked and for fluid to build up in the middle ear. Occasionally, this fluid becomes infected, causing pain and inflammation.

Inner ear

The inner ear contains the most sophisticated part of the hearing mechanism: the fluid-filled, snail-shaped cochlea (KOK-le-uh). The cochlea translates incoming sound waves into signals that can be understood by the brain. See the illustration on page 18.

The spiraling tube of the cochlea would be just over an inch in length if it were stretched out straight, but it naturally curls around almost three times. The whole cochlear structure is no bigger than the size of a pea.

The tube of the cochlea is divided into three chambers that spiral around a bony core. The upper chamber (scala vestibuli) and lower chamber (scala tympani) are filled with a fluid called perilymph. The middle chamber or cochlear duct (scala media) has a different type of fluid called endolymph.

The cochlear duct also contains the organ of Corti, which is vital to the hearing process. Lining the organ of Corti is a strip of tissue called the basilar membrane, on which stand four rows of ultrasensitive hair cells topped by tiny tufts of fine hair strands (cilia). The longest cilia are embedded in an overlying strip of tissue called the tectorial membrane. In response to sound, the hair cells trigger nerve impulses that are transmitted to the brain along the auditory nerve.

The inner ear also contains a structure called the vestibular labyrinth, which assists your sense of balance. It consists of three semicircular tubes that, similar

Inner ear

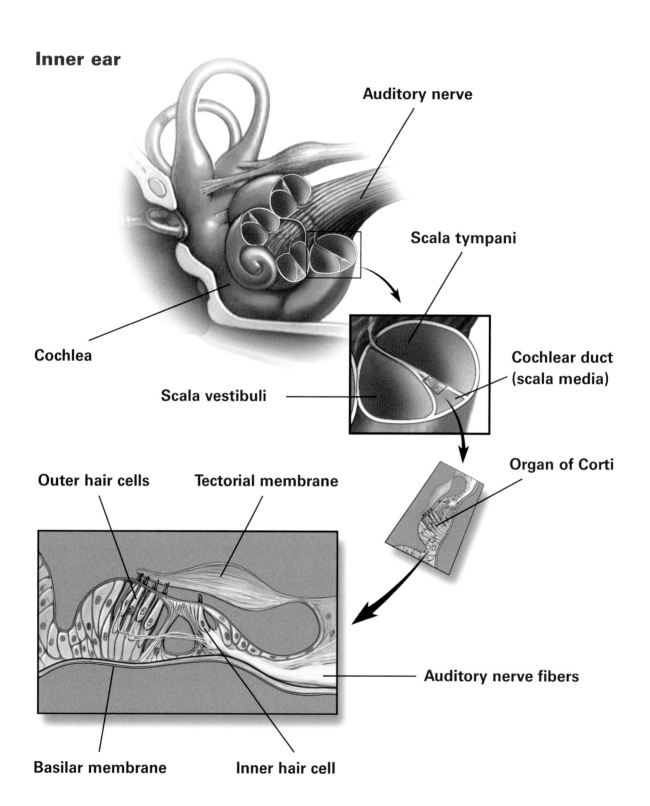

Auditory nerve

Scala tympani

Cochlea

Scala vestibuli

Cochlear duct
(scala media)

Organ of Corti

Outer hair cells

Tectorial membrane

Auditory nerve fibers

Basilar membrane

Inner hair cell

to the cochlea, are filled with fluid and contain hair cells that are sensitive to fluid movement. These cells track every motion of your body to help keep you aware of where your head is in relation to the ground. Chapter 10 describes in greater detail the vestibular labyrinth and symptoms associated with it such as dizziness and vertigo.

Characteristics of sound

The ear is a series of delicate, complex structures that enables you to collect and make sense of sound. But what is sound exactly?

Sound occurs whenever a substance — or rather, the molecules that make up the substance — vibrates. And when a substance vibrates, it displaces all the molecules around it, in much the same way that a rock thrown into a pond causes the water to ripple in every direction. The vibration moves from molecule to molecule in the form of a sound wave.

We hear sound waves that travel through air, such as the clap of an audience's applause at the end of a performance or the hum of pistons and belts in a running car engine.

But sounds also travel through fluid such as water, for example, when you hear the splashes of nearby swimmers when your head's underwater at the pool. Sounds also travel through solid matter such as bone or steel. The thump you hear when you bump your head against an object is partially a result of vibrations traveling through your skull as well as through air.

When a sound wave travels through the air to your outer ear and reaches your eardrum, it triggers a chain reaction through the ossicles, cochlea, auditory nerve and brain that allows you to hear the sound.

As you know, one sound can be vastly different from another. Think of the low-pitched rumble of a diesel truck and the high-pitched whine of a lightweight motorbike. Both sounds come from a combustion engine. But there's no mistaking one sound for the other. The differences between sounds arise mainly from three qualities — frequency, intensity and timbre. The first two qualities can be measured, and the third is subjective.

Frequency

The frequency of sound, a quality also known as pitch, is how often a sound wave fluctuates within a given period of time. This is usually measured in cycles per second, or hertz (Hz). The more fluctuations per second, the higher the frequency.

Sound frequencies audible to humans range from around 20 Hz, a very low pitch, to 20,000 Hz, a very high pitch. Common sounds in human speech cover a broad range from about 250 Hz (a low-pitched vowel such as *ooo*) to around 4,000 Hz (a high-pitched consonant such as *sss*).

Intensity

The intensity of sound is measured by its loudness (amplitude). This quality is associated with the level of disturbance of the sound wave. It's measured in decibels (dB).

For example, a hushed whisper might be measured at 30 decibels sound pressure level (dB SPL), whereas a gunshot might register at 140 to 170 dB SPL. Noise at this intensity is too loud for the human ear to tolerate and can cause permanent damage if the ears aren't protected with earplugs or a hearing protective device (earmuffs).

A subjective description of sound intensity is its loudness. For example, noises can be too soft, comfortably loud, too loud or painfully loud.

Timbre

Perhaps the most subjective aspect of sound is its timbre (TIM-bur), which describes the quality of sound. Timbre allows you to distinguish between sounds of the same frequency and intensity, such as the same note played by different musical instruments or the same consonant or vowel spoken by different voices.

The tone of a piccolo or flute, for example, vibrates within a restricted range of frequencies — it would be represented by a relatively smooth, rolling waveform.

The timbre of a saxophone or piano is more complex — the result of multiple vibrations at many different frequencies — and represented by a jagged waveform. The dissonant ping that results from dropping a wooden pencil on a hard floor is another example of a complex sound.

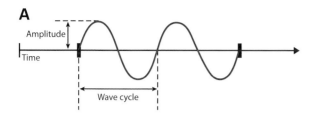

A

Amplitude

Time

Wave cycle

Properties of a sound wave

Amplitude measures how loud a sound is. The number of wave cycles per second measures frequency. The frequency of this sound wave is 2 hertz (Hz) — or two wavelength cycles in one second.

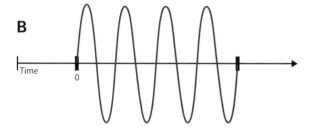

B

Time

0

Sound wave B has a higher frequency and amplitude than does sound wave A, making sound wave B higher pitched and louder.

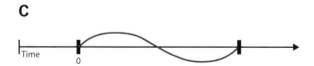

C

Time

0

Sound wave C has a lower frequency and amplitude than does sound wave A, making sound wave C lower pitched and softer — in fact, barely audible.

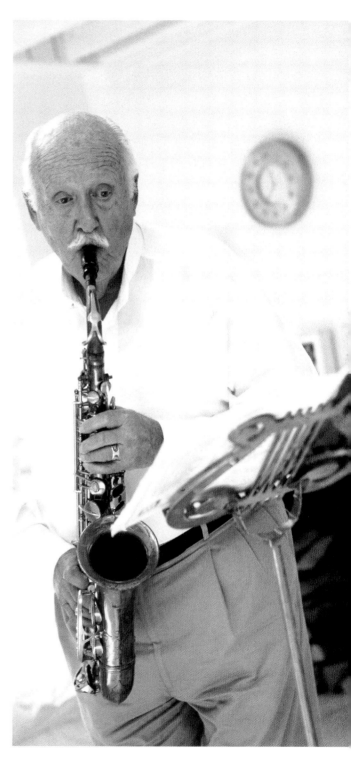

Sound pathways

Sound is created by molecular vibrations moving through matter, and hearing is the perception of that sound. When you hear a sound, you perceive its qualities of frequency, intensity and timbre practically at once. The journey of a sound wave through the ear and to your brain may be almost instantaneous, but it is nonetheless complex.

It begins as the outer ear (pinna) gathers in sound waves and directs them toward your eardrum. Many mammals, such as cats and dogs, have the ability to rotate their outer ears toward the source of a sound. Humans don't have this ability.

Instead, sound waves reach your outer ears from different directions at different angles and at slightly different times and intensities, producing slightly different patterns depending on where the source of a sound is in relation to your head. This helps your brain to locate the source.

Binaural hearing

Hearing with two ears is called binaural hearing — as opposed to monaural hearing with one ear. The use of both ears is critical to helping you locate the source of a sound. A sound occurring on your left will reach your left ear first and register as louder in this ear than in your right. When your brain compares information from both ears, it can distinguish whether the sound has originated from the left or the right.

With the help of auditory information arriving from both ears, your brain is often able to pick out the sounds you want to hear and somewhat suppress the background noise. An example of this function is your ability to hold a conversation with someone at a crowded, noisy party.

Into the middle ear

After a sound wave travels through the ear canal, it strikes the taut membrane of the eardrum, causing the eardrum to vibrate. These vibrations cause the ossicles that bridge the space between the eardrum and the oval window to vibrate also. The ossicles move together like a tiny lever system.

Because the surface of the eardrum is much larger than the oval window, the vibrations are delivered with greater force to the inner ear. Amplifying the

Sound pressure level and hearing level

Decibels are common units of measure that can indicate two different types of sound intensity. Measuring the force of a sound wave in the environment or the amount of pressure it exerts on your eardrum is referred to as sound pressure level. The reference level of 0 decibels sound pressure level (dB SPL) is about the weakest sound that can be heard with the best human ears. The intensity of normal speech is generally around 60 dB SPL.

Decibel units can also establish how well your hearing compares with the average for a large group of young people with normal hearing. This measure is expressed in decibels hearing level (dB HL). A person with a hearing threshold (the faintest level at which he or she can perceive sound) between 0 and 25 dB HL is considered to have normal or near-normal hearing. Someone who has trouble understanding conversations may barely hear sounds at 40 dB HL but not lower, and is considered to have moderate hearing loss. A person who can hear only a loud, nearby voice may have a hearing threshold of 70 dB HL, and is considered to have severe hearing loss.

In subsequent chapters, sound intensity expressed in terms of *dB* will represent a measure of sound pressure level. When referring to a measure of hearing level, it will be expressed as *dB HL.*

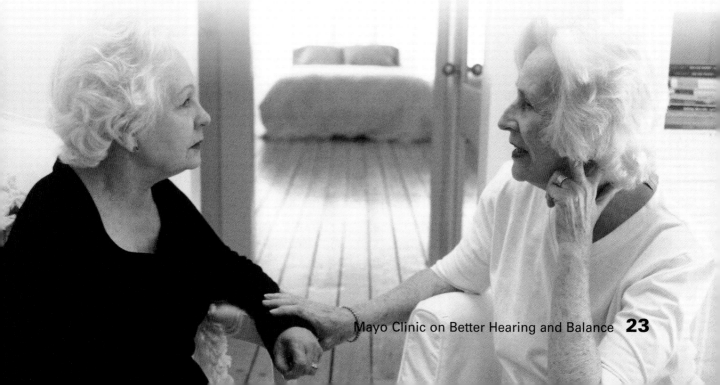

sound increases the energy, which is necessary for the vibrations to travel through the fluid of the inner ear. Fluid offers more resistance than does air and thus requires a greater force to push through it.

If a sound is too loud, muscles in the middle ear constrict to reduce the effects of the sound and protect the inner ear. This is called an acoustic reflex. However, a noise such as a nearby gunshot can cause immediate, permanent damage to the ear. That's because of a slight delay between the auditory nerve's response to a sudden sound and the middle ear muscle's protective contraction. This brief delay leaves the inner ear vulnerable to damage from impact noise.

Into the inner ear

The vibration of the stirrup against the oval window transmits the pattern of the sound wave to the inner ear and the fluid in the upper and lower chambers of the cochlea. The wave sets in motion the hair cells embedded in the basilar membrane (see page 18).

Each frequency of a sound wave affects a specific section of the basilar membrane. This stimulates a response in the

hair cells exactly at that location. If the sound you hear has a very high frequency, the basilar membrane resonates near the base of the cochlea. If the sound wave has a low frequency, the basilar membrane resonates closer to the tip of the cochlea.

This motion displaces the cilia on the hair cells, resulting in a chemical reaction within the hair cells. This chemical reaction triggers electrical impulses in the auditory nerve. The louder or more intense the sound, the more impulses that are sent off.

Traveling to the brain

From the auditory nerve, electrical impulses travel along twin neurological circuits in the brain containing several information-processing stations. These stations start analyzing the signals to determine their origin. For example, the stations for the left ear compare what they've learned with stations for the right ear. This activity also filters background noise. See a visualization of the sound pathways to your brain on pages 26-27.

The neurological circuits end in the auditory cortices, which are located in the temporal lobes on each side of the brain. Arrival of the impulses in the cortices signals the grand finale of the hearing process.

Scientists are still trying to understand how the brain interprets the impulses and identifies them as distinct sounds. At lower frequencies the electrical impulses follow the same pattern as the sound waves. But at high frequencies, this pattern varies.

Speech and language — how the brain gives meaning to sound — is associated closely with your ability to hear. We know that the knowledge and recognition of specific sounds in a person's memory starts at a young age. For example, at about 3 months, babies can differentiate their parents' voices from other voices.

Types of hearing loss

With such a complex auditory system, many small changes or slight damage to the ear can affect some or most of your hearing. Scientists have identified three types of hearing loss: conductive, sensorineural and mixed.

Conductive hearing loss

The ear canal and the middle ear conduct sound waves to the sensory receptors of your inner ear. If something blocks this pathway, the sound waves are disrupted. The result is a reduced perception of sound.

This can occur, for example, from an excessive buildup of wax in the ear canal. Normally, your ear canal cleanses itself, but in some cases buildup occurs and may require professional removal.

Other problems that can cause conductive hearing loss include foreign objects lodged in the ear, middle ear infections, head trauma and abnormal bone growth in the region of the ear. See Chapter 3 for more information about conductive hearing loss.

Sensorineural hearing loss

Damage to the structures of the inner ear, such as the hair cells in the cochlea or the nerve fibers leading from the cochlea to the brain, can cause sensorineural (sen-suh-re-NOOR-ul) hearing loss. Such damage is most often associated with the general wear and

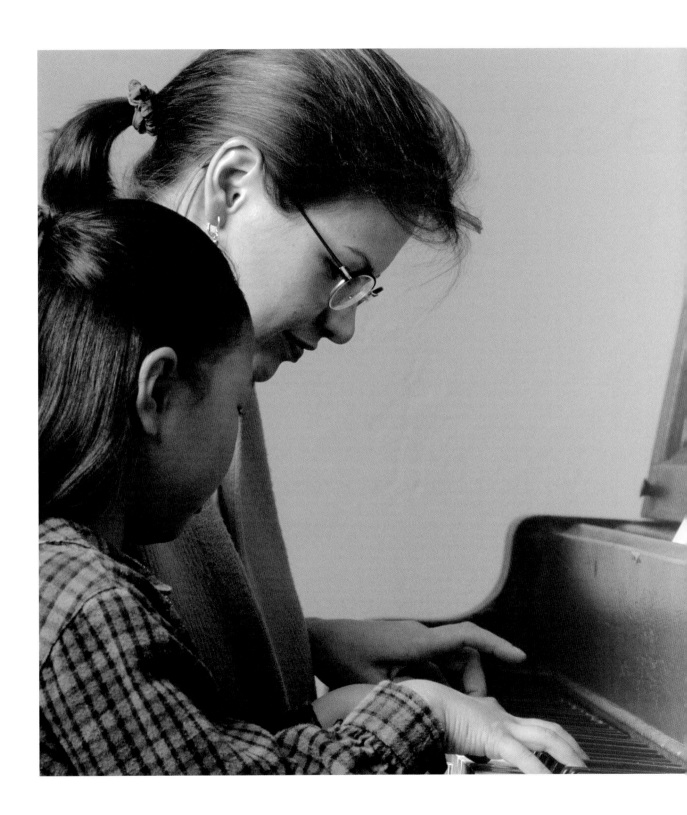

In the ear

Sound waves that have traveled through the ear canal cause the eardrum and ossicles of the middle ear to vibrate. These vibrations trigger a chemical reaction in the cochlea of the inner ear, sending electrical impulses along the auditory nerve and into the brain.

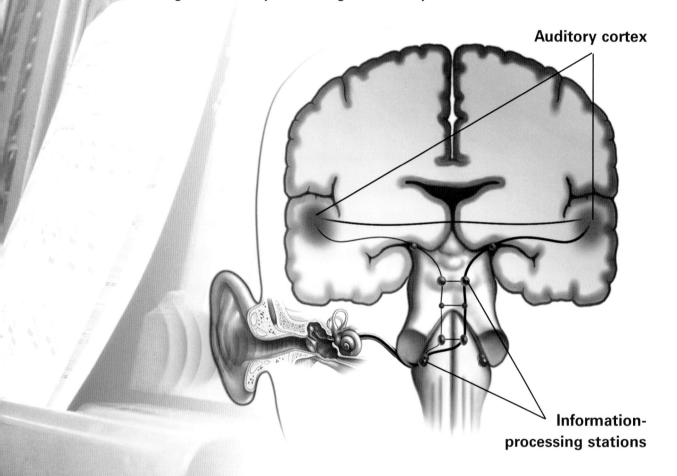

Auditory cortex

Information-processing stations

In the brain

Electrical impulses from the auditory nerve pass through and cross between several information-processing stations on their way to the auditory cortices in the temporal lobes. There, the brain sorts, processes, analyzes, compares and files information about sounds, helping you to make sense of what you hear.

tear of aging, known as presbycusis (pres-bih-KU-sis), or with too much exposure to loud noise.

Initial sensorineural damage is typically found at the base of the cochlea, where the basilar membrane responds

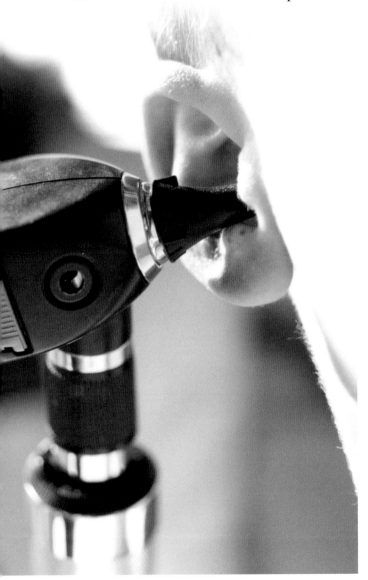

to high frequencies. That's why people with sensorineural hearing loss often have trouble perceiving high-frequency sounds, such as certain consonants used in speech.

For example, someone with high-frequency hearing loss may be unable to distinguish the word *tell* from *sell* or *miff* from *myth*.

Other potential damage to the inner ear may result from high fever or chronic illness, certain powerful medications that can hurt the ear, trauma to the head and genetic disorders. As well, the auditory nerve can be damaged by abnormal growths, such as tumors, and other causes. See Chapter 4 for more information about sensorineural hearing loss.

Mixed hearing loss

Some individuals may have a combination of conductive and sensorineural hearing loss. For example, someone with age-related sensorineural hearing loss may also develop a middle ear infection. The conductive hearing loss caused by the infection can usually be eliminated with medical treatment. However, the sensorineural damage is likely untreatable.

Recognize signs of hearing loss

Look for early signs of hearing loss. The questions below, based on a list from the National Institute on Deafness and Other Communication Disorders, may help you decide whether to see a physician or audiologist for a hearing evaluation. Keep in mind, these general questions may not address everything about your specific situation.

- Do you have a problem with hearing on the telephone?
- Do you have to strain to understand conversation?
- Do you have trouble following a conversation when two or more people are talking at the same time?
- Do you have trouble hearing in a situation with a noisy background?

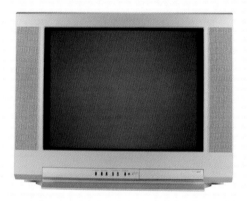

- Do people say that you turn the TV volume up too high?
- Do you find yourself asking people to repeat themselves?
- Do many people you talk to seem to mumble or not speak clearly?
- Do people get annoyed because you misunderstand what they say?
- Do you respond inappropriately to what people say?

- Do you have trouble understanding the speech of people who may have higher pitched voices or are soft spoken — often women and children?

If you answered yes to three or more of these questions, you may think about requesting a hearing evaluation. In addition, ask someone who knows you well to consider these questions with you in mind. He or she might notice signs of hearing loss in you long before you do and prompt you to get help.

Compensating for hearing loss

Hearing loss too often bears the brunt of jokes and comedic skits. Frequently, it's associated with inattention, lower intelligence or just plain "getting old." Some people convince themselves that they don't need to hear everything out there anyway and simply resign themselves to their condition.

But losing some of your hearing can be an obstacle at best and dangerous at worst. Hearing not only helps you to understand what others are saying, but also cues you to where you are and alerts you to danger. Hearing helps you stay connected to the world.

Many people avoid admitting to hearing loss for fear of being stereotyped as someone who consistently misunderstands conversations and talks to others by shouting. They may compensate for their diminished hearing and try to mask it by:
- Asking others to repeat themselves
- Blaming others for mumbling or speaking too softly
- Limiting or withdrawing from social activities

- Turning up the volume on the television or radio
- Smiling and nodding without understanding

If you regularly engage in the actions listed above, you might consider seeking the help of an audiologist to evaluate your hearing.

To deny a real hearing deficit because you don't want others to recognize it is like refusing to look at your shirt in order to detract attention from a stain. Many people will see through your efforts and notice the problem anyway. Addressing a hearing problem can put you on the path to becoming a more active participant in life and a more engaged companion and friend.

Getting a hearing exam

Perhaps you've noticed lately that you have trouble hearing certain letter sounds when someone is talking to you. While attending a lecture recently, you had difficulty distinguishing the speaker's voice from the background noise. Because you're unsure of what's being said, you've become more reluctant to join in conversations.

If these situations are becoming all too familiar, you may be experiencing hearing loss. A hearing exam may help identify the cause and lead to treatment that enables you to hear better and feel more confident socially.

If you want to get your hearing or your child's hearing checked, whom do you see? You might start by talking with your primary physician or your child's pediatrician. Your doctor can do a preliminary hearing exam and provide explanations for many of your concerns. He or she can also refer you to a hearing specialist — an audiologist — if necessary.

In this chapter you'll get a closer look at each of the specialty areas that may be involved in the diagnosis and treatment of hearing loss. You'll also find out when a hearing exam may be necessary, what's involved in the exam and what the results mean. Knowing what tests to expect and why they're performed can help you get the most out of the hearing exam.

Who provides ear care?

Your family doctor may ask about your hearing at medical visits and encourage you to get tested if there are any concerns. In addition, it's wise to talk to your doctor whenever you're routinely exposed to loud noise or notice signs of hearing loss.

Always consult your doctor before buying a hearing aid. Sometimes hearing loss results from wax impaction, infection, tumor or other problems that call for medication or surgery, not a hearing aid. Your doctor can guide you to the most appropriate treatment.

There are different kinds of hearing specialists, primarily otolaryngologists, otologists and audiologists. Because hearing loss may result from a variety of causes, hearing specialists often work closely with specialists in other fields to make a diagnosis and determine the best course of treatment.

Otolaryngologists

Your family doctor may refer you to an otolaryngologist (o-to-lar-ing-GOL-uh-jist) for a hearing examination. Otolaryngologists are medical doctors trained to diagnose and treat diseases of the ears, sinuses, mouth, throat, voice box (larynx) and other structures in the head and neck region. They perform cosmetic and reconstructive surgery of the head and neck. These specialists are also known as otorhinolaryngologists (o-to-ri-no-lar-ing-GOL-uh-jists) or, simply, ear, nose and throat (ENT) physicians.

An otolaryngologist requires broad specialization because these different parts of the head — ears, nose and throat — are interconnected. The ears and throat are joined by the eustachian tubes. The nose and the throat are joined by the nasopharynx. So, what happens in one area can easily affect the other areas. An upper respiratory infection of the sinuses, for example, can spread to the ears or throat.

All otolaryngologists have completed medical school and at least five years of residency, or specialty training. They're also certified by the American Board of Otolaryngology. After their residency, some otolaryngologists pursue an additional one- or two-year fellowship for more extensive training in a chosen specialty.

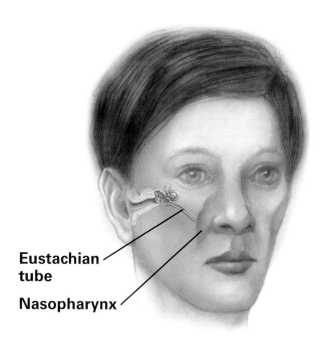

Eustachian tube

Nasopharynx

Ear, nose and throat

An otolaryngologist must have broad specialization because the ears, nose and throat are interconnected.

Otologists

An otologist (o-TOL-uh-jist) is an otolaryngologist who has completed a specialty fellowship focused on ear disorders. Thus, he or she has the most in-depth training devoted to any physical problems of the ear. If your primary doctor suspects that you have an ear disease, you may be referred directly to an otologist.

Some of the conditions that otologists treat include ear infections, facial paralysis, dizziness, hearing loss, ringing in the ears (tinnitus), tumors and congenital deformities. If you need surgery for an ear disorder, you'll probably see an otologist or an otolaryngologist with special training in ear surgery.

Audiologists

An audiologist (aw-de-OL-uh-jist) is trained to evaluate the perceptual aspects of your hearing. If you complain of hearing loss but your doctor finds no physical signs of disease, you may be referred to an audiologist. The audiologist can assess the type of hearing loss you have and measure its severity. Audiologists also evaluate and fit hearing aids and help with hearing rehabilitation.

Audiologists hold a master's degree or doctoral degree in audiology and must have completed an externship — one year of on-the-job experience — before they're able to practice independently. They're certified by the American Speech-Language-Hearing Association (ASHA) or the American Academy of Audiology (AAA). All states require audiologists to be licensed in the state in which they practice.

Working together

Often, these different specialists work together to diagnose and treat a condition. For example, your otologist may refer you to an audiologist to have your hearing tested before treating an ear disorder, and again later to see if the treatment is having an effect.

In contrast, an audiologist may be evaluating you and suspect that your hearing loss is due to a medical problem. In that case, you'll likely be referred to an otologist or otolaryngologist for treatment. Subsequently, the audiologist may see you again for hearing rehabilitation. The sequence of visits is important because each specialist approaches the problem with different training and from a different perspective.

In addition, audiologists may monitor the hearing of individuals who are undergoing treatment for an illness such as cancer or an infectious disease. Some chemotherapy and antibiotic drugs can damage a person's hearing, so the oncologist or infectious disease specialist will work closely with an audiologist to monitor the person's hearing and, if possible, keep the prescribed drug dosage low enough to avoid auditory damage.

Schedule for hearing exams

Everyone should have their hearing tested, from newborns to older adults. An exam can be performed on request if you're concerned about hearing loss or when situations occur that increase your risk of hearing loss. Sometimes the exam is mandated by law.

Children

The screening of newborns is now a common practice in most hospitals in the United States. In fact, in most states testing is mandatory. That's because each year more than 4,000 babies are born with some hearing impairment. Failure to identify the impairment early enough can lead to delayed speech and language development.

Children with unidentified hearing loss often don't do as well in school as their peers do. They're also more likely to be held back a grade or drop out. Because hearing loss isn't readily noticeable, adults may attribute a child's perceived inattention to other causes, such as being distracted or lazy. Early treatment can help prevent many of the

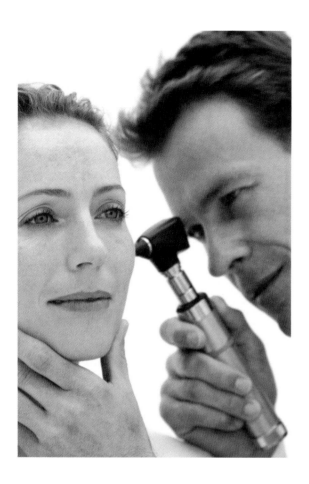

In addition, babies considered to be at high risk of hearing loss should be screened regularly. This group includes infants with a medical history of:

- Severe oxygen deprivation at birth (birth asphyxia)
- Exposure in the womb to an infection such as German measles (rubella) or syphilis
- Exposure to herpes during passage through the birth canal
- Infection such as bacterial meningitis
- Severe jaundice
- Head trauma
- Nervous system disorder associated with hearing loss
- Chronic ear infection
- Family history of hearing loss during childhood

Adults

Screening for adults is not done on a regular schedule. Generally, it's performed at their request. ASHA recommends that adults get their hearing checked every 10 years through age 50 and every three years after that.

Hearing loss increases with age — 14 percent of individuals between 45 and 64 years of age have some degree of hearing loss. That jumps to 30 percent for individuals age 65 or older.

problems related to hearing loss and provide the child with the necessary tools to be successful at school.

Some types of hearing loss in children don't develop until months or years after birth, so periodic screening is recommended during the infant and toddler stages and throughout the school years. See pages 36-37 for the recommended screening schedules.

Recommended screening schedules

Infants

- Initial screening by 1 month of age, preferably at birth.
- If indicated by initial screening, further evaluation to confirm hearing loss by 3 months of age.
- Initiate appropriate treatment for infants with hearing loss before 6 months of age. Ongoing monitoring every three months.
- Screen children deemed to be at high risk of hearing loss every six months until age 3.

School-age children

- On first entry into school system.
- Annually from kindergarten through 3rd grade.
- At 7th grade.
- At 11th grade.
- On entry to special education.
- On repeating a grade.
- On entry to a new school system without evidence of previous screening.
- When indicated by parent or caregiver, by medical or school concern, or by high-risk factors of hearing loss.

Adults

- Every 10 years through age 50 and every three years thereafter.

Employees

- Before employment.
- Before assignment to a hearing-hazardous work area.[*]
- Annually while assigned to a hearing-hazardous work area.
- After ending assignment to a hearing-hazardous work area.
- At termination of employment.

[*]A hearing-hazardous work area is considered an environment with noise exposure equal to or greater than 85 decibels, if averaged over eight hours.

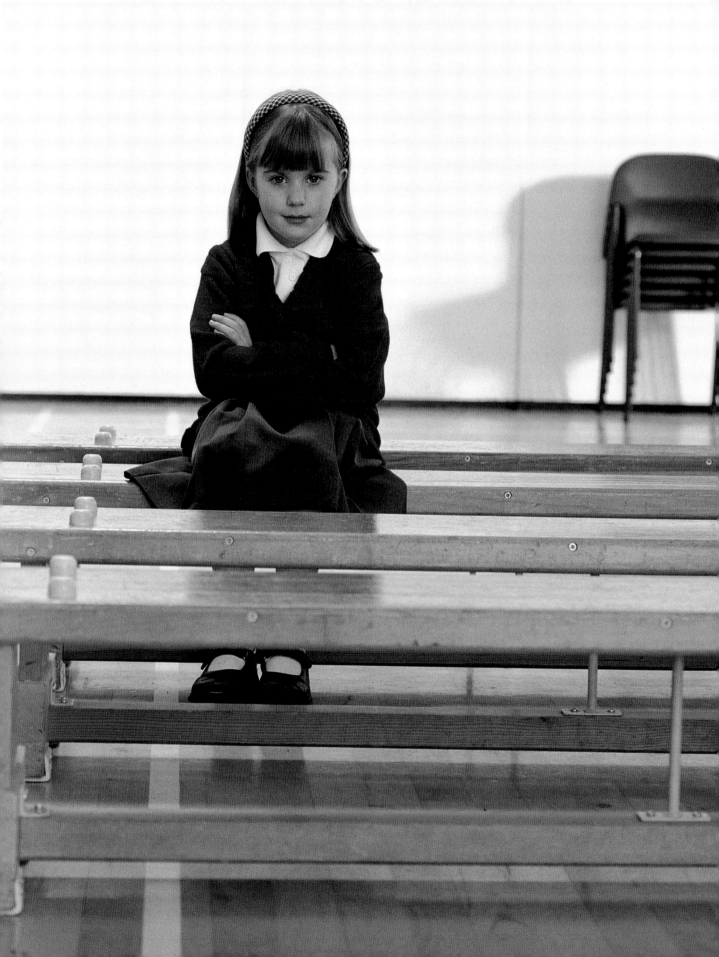

Employees

Prolonged exposure to loud noise can cause gradual, and often permanent, hearing loss. The Occupational Safety and Health Administration (OSHA) requires that employers monitor their companies for noise levels at 85 decibels (dB) or above, averaged over eight working hours.

Under such conditions the employer must develop and maintain a hearing conservation program at no cost to the employee. The program would include regular hearing exams, noise monitoring, access to earplugs or protective devices such as earmuffs, record keeping and employee training regarding hearing protection.

If regular screening indicates hearing loss has occurred, the employee must be informed and wear hearing protectors in work environments with noise levels of 85 dB or more. Hearing protectors are required for all employees when noise levels exceed 90 dB, if the levels are averaged over eight hours.

In order for hearing protectors to be effective, it's important that they fit properly and are worn continuously during periods of noise exposure.

OSHA requires that a qualified hearing specialist administer the program.

Typical hearing exam

A physician and an audiologist will complete different portions of a hearing examination in order to assess all aspects of your hearing. If there's evidence of hearing loss, they will evaluate the signs and symptoms and check for other medical conditions that may be causing the problem. This will help them to determine the severity of your hearing loss and suggest an appropriate course of treatment.

The tests will involve an overall medical evaluation that includes a medical history, physical examination of your ears and laboratory tests. Audiological exams include audiometry, speech reception and word recognition, as well as other tests.

Medical evaluation

The first step in your hearing exam, whether you consult your family doctor or an ear specialist, is to get a full medical evaluation. This helps the doctor determine your overall health status and whether your hearing loss could be the result of an underlying syndrome or disease. The medical evaluation generally includes some or all of the following components:

Medical history. Your examiner will want to fully document the development of your hearing problem. You'll need to be ready for many questions.

- When did you first become aware of the signs and symptoms of hearing loss?
- Is the impairment in one ear or are both ears affected?
- Is the problem getting worse, improving or staying the same?
- Are some sounds more difficult to hear than other sounds, or are all sounds equally hard to distinguish?
- Do you have difficulty recognizing where a sound comes from?
- Are you experiencing signs and symptoms such as ear pain, discharge, infection, dizziness, ringing in the ears and loss of balance?
- Do any members of your family have hearing problems?

Be sure to tell your examiner if you've had long exposure to loud noise, either at work or home. In addition, tell the

doctor if you've ever experienced head trauma, ear surgery or chronic illness, or whether you've recently had an upper respiratory infection, such as a cold or pneumonia. Let your examiner know what medications you're taking or have recently taken.

Physical exam. The next part of your exam will be to examine the size, shape and position of your outer ear (pinna) and to inspect it for any swelling, deformity or redness. This step may yield information about other problems that may be causing hearing loss.

Your examiner may check your eyes, nasal cavity, mouth and neck for any problems that might be associated with ear damage. A slender, flexible tube with a light at the end is used to check for signs of fluid buildup or infection in the back of your nose and upper throat (nasopharynx) and your eustachian tubes, which connect your ears to your nasopharynx.

Otoscopy. The examination of the ear canal, eardrum and middle ear is called an otoscopy — the prefix *oto-* simply refers to "ear." For the test, your physician or audiologist typically uses an instrument called an otoscope, which contains a light and magnifying lens. A

Otoscope

This device illuminates and magnifies the ear canal, eardrum and middle ear, helping the physician to assess your ear health and check for abnormalities.

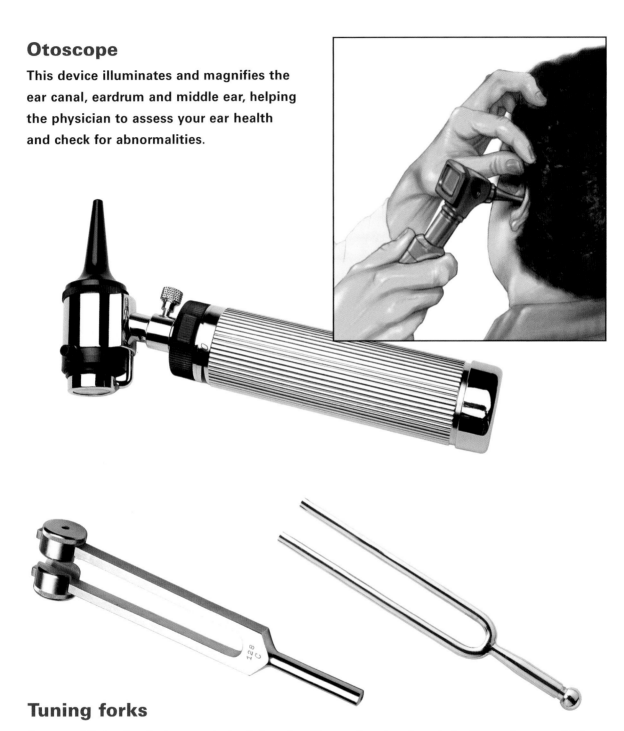

Tuning forks

A test with tuning forks may help determine if your hearing loss is in the outer or middle ear (conductive) or in the inner ear (sensorineural).

specially designed microscope, called an otomicroscope, may also be used to view the ear canal and eardrum.

Generally, an otoscopic examination takes a minute or two and is painless. The examiner may look for wax or fluid buildup, foreign objects, a tumor or skin abnormalities in the ear canal, and any small tears or perforations in the eardrum. He or she also notes whether the eardrum is translucent and has its normal pearly gray color. A bulging eardrum membrane may indicate fluid in the middle ear.

Tuning fork test. A tuning fork looks like a dining fork with only two tines. Made of steel, it sounds a single tone when struck against a solid object — and that tone varies according to the shape and thickness of the tines.

To conduct the test, vibrating forks with different pitches are positioned near your ear to measure your hearing sensitivity to the air conduction of sound waves. The forks are also placed against your skull to measure your sensitivity to the bone conduction of sound waves.

Comparing the results of these tests provides important clues to the cause

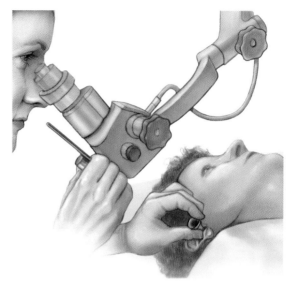

Otomicroscope

An otomicroscope provides a more detailed look into your ear. The physician gently inserts a small viewing funnel into your ear canal to focus the image.

of your hearing loss. People whose hearing is reduced by air conduction but is normal by bone conduction typically have conductive hearing loss — sound waves have difficulty passing through the ear canal or middle ear. People whose hearing is reduced both by air conduction and bone conduction generally have sensorineural hearing loss due to damage in the inner ear.

Laboratory tests. Your physician may request certain blood tests to confirm or rule out possible infectious or inflammatory diseases that are associated with hearing loss. These include syphilis, German measles (rubella), cytomegalovirus — a gastrointestinal infection — and several autoimmune disorders.

These blood tests are particularly important for pregnant women. One of these diseases in an expectant mother can lead to hearing loss that's present at birth (congenital) in her baby. Blood samples also may be examined for DNA abnormalities.

Imaging tests. If your physician suspects that a tumor, tissue abnormality or damage to the auditory nerve is the cause of your hearing loss, a request may be made for detailed images of the interior of your head. Technology to produce these images includes magnetic resonance imaging (MRI) and computerized tomography (CT).

MRI technology creates detailed images of soft tissues using magnetic fields and radio waves. CT technology produces images of bone structure from a series of X-rays. Both types of imaging can reveal a variety of disorders that would otherwise remain unseen, helping lead to a correct diagnosis. Sophisticated imaging technology may also be used to locate congenital abnormalities and trauma-related damage to the ear.

Audiological exams

The audiological exam is focused on hearing function — how well you hear — rather than on physical signs of disease. Audiologists use various tests to determine your hearing status and degree of hearing loss.

These tests can help distinguish between different types of possible hearing loss, reveal whether the impairment is in one or both ears, and determine whether the hearing loss involves one, two or more frequencies. Repeat testing can gauge whether the impairment is getting worse.

These exams are usually conducted using electronic equipment and a room designed to muffle sound so that background noise doesn't interfere.

Audiometry. This testing measures your ability to hear pure tones, such as a middle C and higher notes, through air and through bone. The previously described tuning fork test is a rudimentary form of the audiometric test.

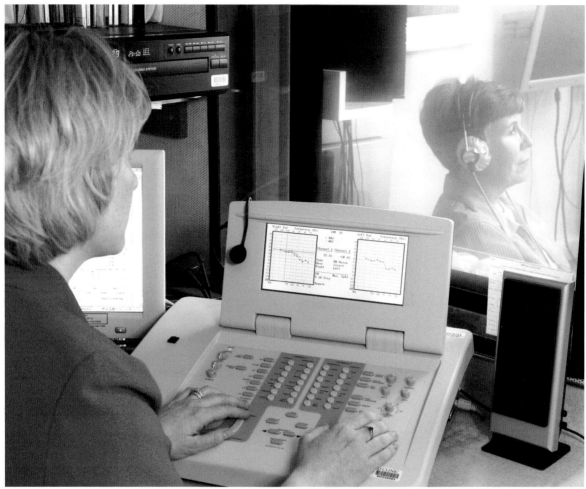

Audiometry

During audiometry, you'll be seated in a sound-treated room (top right in photograph) separate from the audiologist. You'll signal the audiologist whenever you hear a tone played through the earphones. Your hearing thresholds at different pitches will be recorded on an audiogram (graph on the left of screen shot). Also displayed are the results of tympanometry, acoustic reflex and speech recognition.

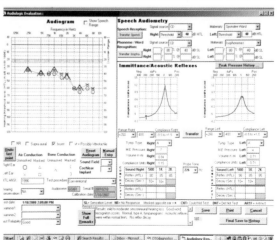

Levels of hearing loss

Decibel (dB) range	Level of hearing loss	Characteristics
16 to 25 dB HL	Slight to minimal	• Has difficulty hearing faint or distant sounds
26 to 30 dB HL	Mild	• Occasionally misses consonants • Has increasing difficulty in understanding with noisy backgrounds and faraway speakers
31 to 50 dB HL	Moderate	• Can understand normal conversation if face to face and vocabulary is controlled
51 to 70 dB HL	Moderate to severe	• May miss most of what's said in a normal conversation • Has difficulty listening in a group setting
71 to 90 dB HL	Severe	• May not be able to hear speech unless very loud • Needs amplification to be able to converse normally
91 dB HL and above	Profound	• May not be able to hear speech at all • Relies on visual cues such as lip reading or sign language

Source: American Speech-Language-Hearing Association, 2003

To check your hearing by way of air conduction, the examiner places earphones over your ears or small, soft tips into your ear canals. Certain tones are introduced through the earphones to one ear at a time.

By varying the frequency and intensity of the tones, the examiner determines the faintest sounds you can hear — known as hearing thresholds. You'll be directed to signal, usually by raising a hand or pressing a button, whenever you hear a tone. Your responses are recorded on a type of graph called an audiogram.

Checking your hearing for sounds conducted through the bones of your skull can help locate problems in the outer and middle ear. To do this the examiner places a special vibrating device either behind your ear or on your forehead. The vibrations travel through your skull, thus bypassing any blockage that may be present in the outer or middle ear.

If test results show that you hear sound when it's conducted through skull bone better than through the air- or fluid-filled passageways in your ear, then sound isn't getting through the outer ear and middle ear properly. It's likely that you have some form of conductive hearing loss. If results show that your hearing is no better via bone conduction than through air conduction, it's likely to be a sensorineural problem with the inner ear.

Speech reception test. For this test, the audiologist plays a recording of, or speaks, familiar two-syllable words, such as *pancake* or *baseball*, while you listen through headphones. Each syllable of a spoken word is pronounced with equal emphasis.

As you hear a word, you repeat it or point to a picture of it. The intensity of the words gradually softens. The faintest level of speech you can understand at least half the time is called your speech reception threshold (SRT).

If your SRT is normal — typically in a range between 0 and 25 decibels, or dB — you should not have difficulty hearing and should be able to understand conversational speech in a quiet environment. If your SRT is 26 dB or higher, you're experiencing progressively more severe levels of hearing loss. A SRT greater than 91 dB indicates profound hearing loss. Generally, there's a strong correlation between the SRT and your audiometry test results.

Word recognition test. This test, also known as a speech discrimination test, determines how well you can understand speech at a comfortable volume — typically set at about 40 dB above your SRT level. (Remember that the SRT is a threshold below which sounds are inaudible to you.)

For the test, you must identify a series of familiar single-syllable words such as *come, thin, sack* and *knees*. When you hear the words, either from a recording or spoken, at a constant, steady volume, you repeat each word or point to a picture of it. Occasionally, background noise is added to see how distraction might affect your understanding.

Your score reflects the percentage of words you've identified correctly. A score between 90 percent and 100 percent means you should have little difficulty understanding conversation. A score of 60 percent to 69 percent indicates that you're having difficulty, and less than 40 percent means extreme difficulty in understanding speech.

Word recognition performed with and without a hearing aid indicates how helpful the device can be to you, and guide your decision about whether or not to use one.

Other tests

In addition to the medical evaluation and audiological exam, your doctor or audiologist may wish to test other aspects of your hearing. These tests can help to refine the diagnosis or determine which treatment options would be most beneficial to you. The additional tests include:

Tympanometry. This test is used to check the function of your eardrum and middle ear. Tympanometry (tim-puh-NOM-uh-tre) helps detect conditions such as a perforated eardrum, fluid in the middle ear and reduced air pressure in the middle ear resulting in a retraction of the eardrum.

To conduct the test, your examiner places a soft probe in your ear canal. As small, varying amounts of air pressure are directed toward your ear, the device measures the corresponding movements of your eardrum. The results are charted on a graph called a tympanogram.

Normal response produces a line rising to a sharp peak in the middle of the tympanogram. But if fluid is in the middle ear, the eardrum doesn't move easily and the graph's line doesn't

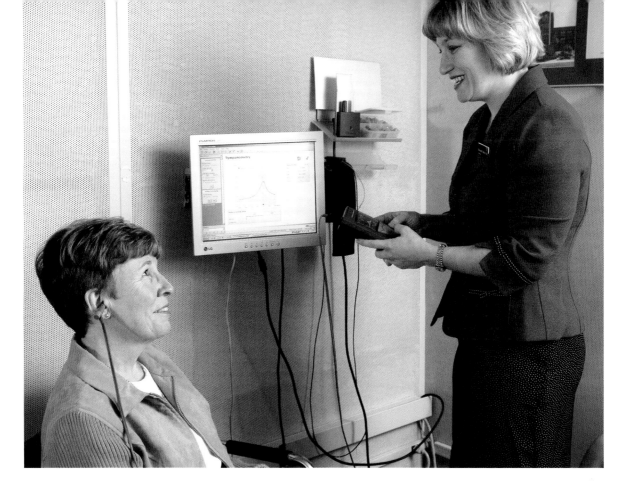

Tympanometry

This test records the response of your eardrum to varying amounts of air pressure. The tympanogram can indicate conductive problems such as a perforated eardrum or fluid buildup in the middle ear.

peak. The graph can also reveal whether the air pressure in the middle ear is less than or greater than outside atmospheric pressure.

Acoustic reflex test. An acoustic reflex test measures the level at which the muscle in your middle ear contracts in response to sounds that are too loud.

The acoustic reflex is described on page 24 in Chapter 1.

During the test you hear sounds at varying levels of intensity. The level at which the reflex contraction occurs, or the absence of reflex, helps evaluate your hearing loss and locate problems along the auditory pathway.

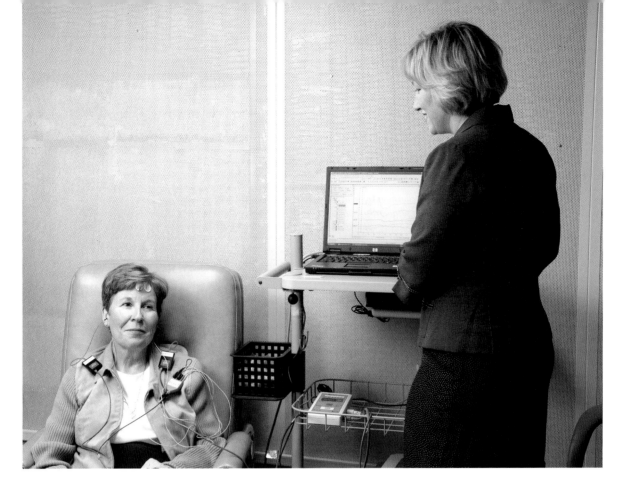

Auditory brainstem response

Electrodes attached to your ears and head measure how the auditory nerve receives electrical impulses from the inner ear and transmits them to the brain.

Auditory brainstem response test. This test measures the electrical nerve impulses sent from the inner ear to the brain when sounds are introduced to the ear. Electrodes are placed in the ear canal or around the ear as well as on your head. Earphones introduce a series of short clicking sounds to your ear. A computer hooked up to the electrodes records neurological activity as the auditory nerve transmits the impulses to the brain.

Because this test doesn't require a voluntary response, such as a hand signal, from the person being tested, it's often used to screen hearing in newborns and infants. This test can be used to assess other problems with the auditory nerve.

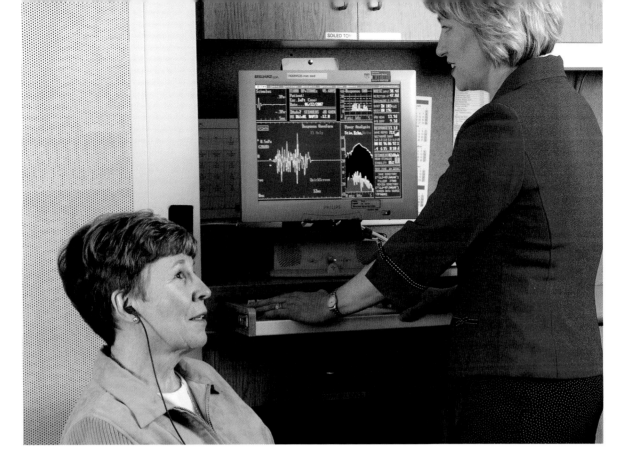

Otoacoustic emissions

A probe with a small microphone is placed in your ear canal to check for otoacoustic emissions. These inaudible echoes are produced in people with normal hearing but not in people with hearing loss — thus, if a test doesn't register them, there's a hearing problem.

Otoacoustic emissions test. This test measures an interesting phenomenon that occurs in hair cells of your inner ear. These cells respond to the movement of fluid in the cochlea. The resulting vibrations of the hair cells produce inaudible sounds called otoacoustic emissions. These emissions can be measured by placing a probe equipped with a microphone into the ear canal.

This test is useful because people with normal hearing produce otoacoustic emissions, but people with hearing loss caused by damaged hair cells don't produce them. Test results help the examiner assess the degree of loss.

This test is also used to screen hearing in newborns and infants because it doesn't require a voluntary response.

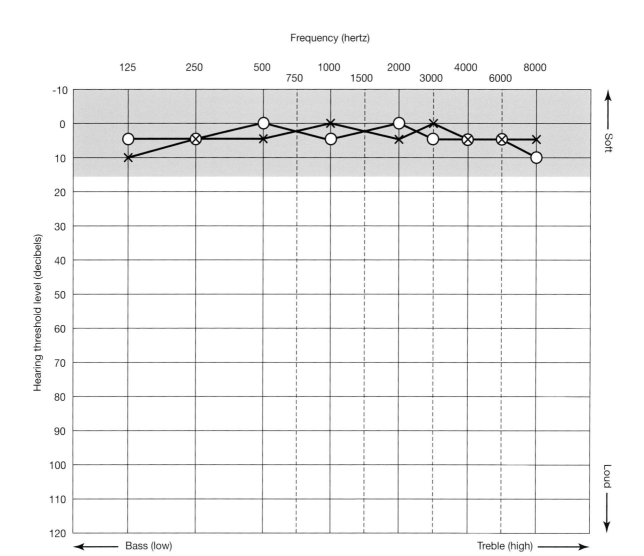

Frequency (hertz)

O Right ear X Left ear Range of normal hearing

Audiogram for normal hearing

This audiogram shows normal hearing in both the right ear and the left ear. Hearing in the right ear is plotted with Os and in the left ear with Xs. If your hearing is normal, all your Xs and Os will typically fall in the range between −10 decibels hearing level (dB HL) and 15 dB HL (shaded area on the audiogram). As hearing loss develops, the Xs and Os fall lower and lower on the graph, and below the shaded area.

Understanding your audiogram

Your physician or audiologist may use any or all of the tests described in the previous section to compile a detailed assessment of your hearing. But the test that's relied on most is audiometry. The resulting graph, the audiogram, is a baseline indicator of your hearing. The graph reveals the softest sounds you can hear at different pitches.

At first glance an audiogram may seem baffling. To understand what the lines and numbers represent, it's helpful to look at each component of the graph separately.

The audiogram portrays sound in terms of two of its most important qualities: frequency (pitch) measured in hertz, and intensity (loudness) measured in decibels.

The vertical lines represent the range of frequencies, which moves from a bass or low pitch on the left (125 Hz) to a treble or high pitch on the right (8,000 Hz). The frequencies most common in human speech are between 500 Hz and 4,000 Hz. Some speech sounds have a very low pitch, such as *vv* in vacuum or *mm* in morning. Speech sounds such as *ff* in food and *th* in thanks have a high pitch.

The horizontal lines on the audiogram represent how loud the sound is. These levels range from -10 dB at the top of the graph (soft) to 120 dB at the bottom (loud). Zero dB represents very faint sounds that someone with normal hearing can generally hear.

Every point on an audiogram represents a different sound, determined by its pitch at a given intensity. When you take an audiometric test, your response to the different sounds you hear are recorded on the graph. At each frequency, the faintest tone that you can hear in your right ear is recorded as an O and the faintest tone you can hear in your left ear is recorded as an X. The resulting lines of Os and Xs on the graph represent hearing thresholds for your ears — any softer sounds are inaudible to you.

Some people may have symmetrical hearing loss, which means the thresholds are approximately at the same level in both ears. Others may have asymmetrical hearing loss, which means one ear has a higher threshold

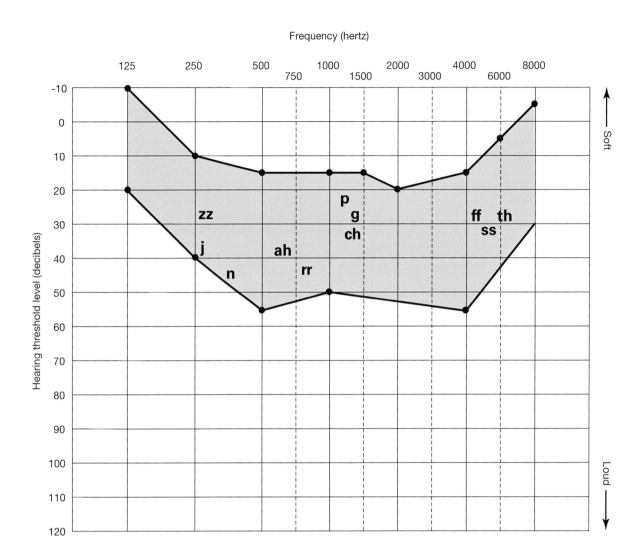

Speech spectrum

The shaded portion of this audiogram indicates the speech spectrum. This shows the irregular concave arc where the sounds of normal human speech lie. Softer, high-pitched sounds such as *ff*, *th* and *ss* appear on the right-hand side of the audiogram. Louder, low-pitched sounds such as *zz* and the letters *j* and *n* appear on the left-hand side.

than the other. Hearing loss may vary according to frequency. For example, someone may have normal hearing at low and middle frequencies in both ears. But he or she may have moderate to severe loss at high frequencies in the left ear and only mild loss at high frequencies in the right ear.

The speech spectrum

If the audiogram represented all of the sounds that make up human speech at a normal conversational level, it would show up as a concave-shaped — or banana-shaped — area just above the middle of the graph. This area is known as the speech spectrum. Soft, high-pitched sounds such as *ss, ff* and *th* would be in the right-hand portion of the spectrum. Loud, low-pitched sounds such as *zz, jj* and *nn* would appear in the left-hand portion. Sounds such as *ch* and *gg* fall somewhere in between.

If the graph showed the speech spectrum superimposed over your audiometric test results, you would have a visual representation of which portions

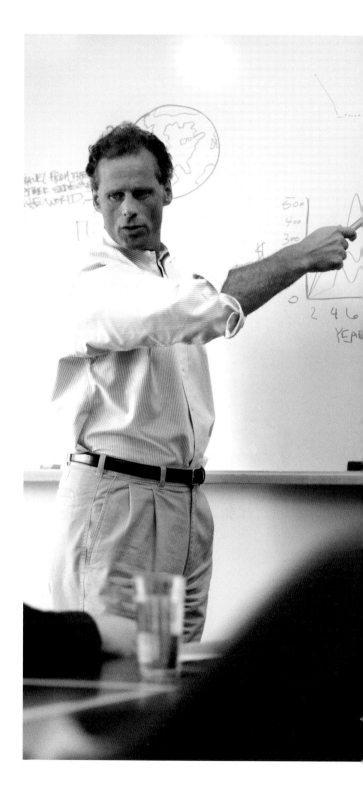

of conversational speech are audible to you and which are inaudible. The inaudible sounds could be heard only if the decibel level were increased and the sounds made louder.

Sometimes you don't think about getting your hearing checked until you notice that something is obviously wrong or another person calls a hearing problem to your attention. Hearing loss may be tough to admit to and is often viewed as a sign of old age.

But protecting your hearing can have an immediate and positive physical, social and emotional impact on your life. Treatment may help eliminate feelings of isolation and frustration and allow you to participate more actively in the world around you. A decision to take action today and schedule a hearing exam can determine how well you'll be hearing in the weeks, months and years ahead.

Problems of the outer ear and middle ear

A primary function of both the outer ear and the middle ear is to direct — or conduct — sound waves to the sensitive auditory structures of the inner ear. This function allows strong, clear signals to be processed by the brain into sounds that you can make sense of and recognize.

Conductive hearing loss occurs when something interferes with the passage of sound waves through the outer ear and middle ear — very often, the function of the inner ear is normal. When you have conductive hearing loss, all sounds that you hear, no matter the frequency (pitch) or intensity (loudness), seem muffled. What are soft or faint sounds to someone with normal hearing become inaudible to you.

A number of problems can obstruct the sound waves on their passage to the inner ear. The problems may include too much earwax, ruptured eardrum or infection that causes a fluid buildup in your middle ear.

Often, conductive hearing loss can be reversed with proper treatment, sometimes involving self-care and sometimes requiring medication or surgery.

Problems of the outer ear and middle ear generally don't cause permanent damage. This chapter describes many of the common causes of conductive hearing loss and guidelines for treating these conditions.

Outer ear problems

Problems that occur in your outer ear are more often a discomfort and annoyance than a serious medical condition. With proper self-care and, if necessary, treatment from a doctor, outer ear problems usually can be resolved and your hearing restored to its normal level. The most common outer ear problems include earwax blockage, a foreign object lodged in the ear and swimmer's ear.

Earwax blockage

The skin lining the outer portion of your ear canal contains glands that produce a waxy substance called cerumen, more commonly known as earwax. This wax is part of your body's normal defense against harm. It traps dust and other foreign particles that collect in the outer ear to keep them from injuring the delicate eardrum (tympanic membrane). Wax also helps inhibit the growth of bacteria.

Normally, earwax migrates to the outer edge of the ear canal and either falls out or is wiped away when you clean your outer ear. At times you may produce more wax than your ear can expel, causing the wax to accumulate in your ear canal.

Generally, an excess amount of earwax doesn't lead to hearing loss because it doesn't completely block the passageway. But many people insert objects such as cotton swabs, hairpins, keys and even a finger into the ear canal, presumably to clean it. These actions push the wax farther into the passageway and impact it. Impacted earwax, as it builds, can reduce your hearing by blocking airborne sound vibrations in your ear canal.

Blockage can make your ear feel full or plugged. Rarely, it can cause noise such as ringing, buzzing or roaring in your ears (tinnitus).

Treatment. To remove excess wax from your ears, you may consult a doctor or try the following self-care method:

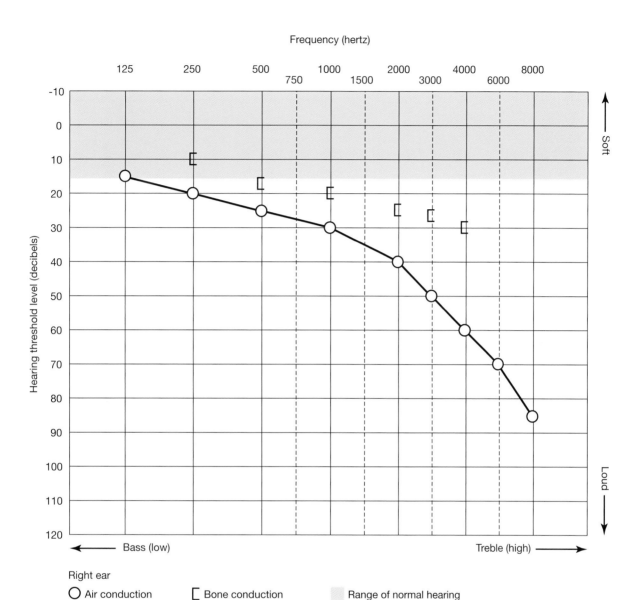

Frequency (hertz)

Hearing threshold level (decibels)

Soft

Loud

← Bass (low)

Treble (high) →

Right ear

○ Air conduction   ⌷ Bone conduction   ▒ Range of normal hearing

Hearing loss due to earwax blockage

This audiogram shows a typical pattern of hearing loss due to earwax blockage in the right ear. Results show increasing difficulty in hearing sounds at higher frequencies. You would need sounds at 6,000 hertz to be at least 70 decibels HL in order to hear them.

- Soften the earwax with a few drops of baby oil, mineral oil or olive oil from an eyedropper twice a day for several days.
- When the wax is softened, fill a bowl with water heated to body temperature — if the water is colder or hotter than body temperature, application may make you feel dizzy during the procedure.
- With your head upright, grasp the top of your ear and pull upward. With your other hand, squirt water gently into your ear canal with a 3-ounce rubber-bulb syringe. Lower your head to the side and allow the water to drain into the bowl.
- You may need to repeat the previous step several times before the excess wax falls out.
- Dry your ear carefully with a towel or hand-held hair dryer. Insert a few drops of an alcohol-vinegar preparation (half rubbing alcohol, half white vinegar) with an eye-dropper to help dry your ear.

Earwax removers sold in stores (Murine, others) also can be effective. One note of caution: If you've previously ruptured an eardrum or had ear surgery, don't flush your ears unless your doctor approves. Such action could lead to pain or infection.

If after self-care you still have excess wax in your ears, seek the help of your doctor. He or she may repeat the washing of your ears or use special instruments to either scoop or suction out the impacted earwax.

Foreign object in the ear

Occasionally, an object such as a piece of cotton thread from a swab, a bit of paper, an earplug or even an insect can become stuck in your ear. You may notice this when your ear begins to tickle, hurt or feel plugged.

Most foreign objects lodge in the ear canal and don't cause lasting hearing problems. But if an object is pushed too far into your ear, it may rupture your eardrum and potentially damage your middle ear, which can have more serious consequences.

Treatment. Here's advice for occasions when a foreign object becomes lodged in your ear:
- Don't attempt to remove the foreign object by probing with a cotton swab, matchstick or any other tool. To do so is to risk pushing the object farther into the ear, making it harder to extract and possibly causing more serious damage.

- You may be able to dislodge the object by tilting your head toward the affected side and shaking it gently in the direction of the ground.
- If the object is clearly visible to an observer, is pliable and can be grasped easily with tweezers, he or she may be able to gently remove it.
- If the object isn't accessible, contact your doctor or a hospital emergency room. The doctor will need to remove the object with tiny forceps or suction or by flooding it out with fluid. He or she can check to see if any damage has occurred.
- If an insect is lodged in the ear and is still alive, tilt the affected ear upward. Insects instinctively crawl up, rather than down, in order to free themselves.
- If the insect doesn't exit the ear on its own, place a few drops of warm — not hot — baby oil, mineral oil or olive oil into the ear. You can ease the entry of the oil by gently pulling the top of the ear back and upward. The insect should suffocate and float out in the oil bath.
- Don't use oil to remove objects other than an insect. Also, don't apply oil if any of the signs or symptoms of a perforated eardrum are present, such as pain, bleeding or discharge from the ear.

Swimmer's ear

Swimmer's ear (otitis externa) is an infection of the ear canal. Usually, it's the result of persistent moisture in the ear — for example, frequent swimming — often in combination with a mild injury to the skin of the ear canal.

This condition can result from scraping the ear canal to clean out wax. This creates ideal circumstances for bacteria and fungi to invade the ear canal and cause infection. Hair spray and hair dyes also may cause infection or allergic reaction. Swimmer's ear is most common in children and young adults.

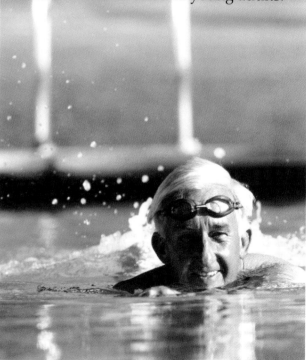

Pain or itching in the ear, a swollen ear canal and the drainage of pus are signs and symptoms of an outer ear infection. Temporary hearing loss may occur if the swelling or pus blocks the ear canal.

Treatment. If the pain is mild and you don't have ear drainage or hearing loss, follow the self-care tips below. Otherwise, seek medical attention.

- Place a warm — not hot — heating pad over your ear. But don't lie on the heating pad.
- Consider taking a pain reliever such as ibuprofen (Advil, Motrin, others) or acetaminophen (Tylenol, others), if needed.
- Keep water, fluids and other substances out of your ear canal while it's healing.
- Place a few drops of an alcohol-vinegar preparation (half rubbing alcohol, half white vinegar) in your ear after showering or swimming. The alcohol helps keep the skin of your ear canal dry, and the vinegar helps prevent bacterial and fungal growth from occurring.

Over-the-counter ear-water drying drops also are available for use after swimming (Auro-Dri, Swim-Ear, others). These are easy to use.

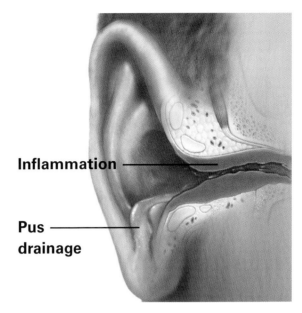

Inflammation

Pus drainage

Outer ear infection

A small cut allows bacteria and fungi to invade the ear canal and cause infection.

If the ear pain doesn't subside after a day or two, or if you have additional concerns, see your doctor. After cleaning your ear, the doctor may prescribe eardrops containing a corticosteroid to relieve itching and decrease inflammation, and antibiotics to control infection. More severe infections may be treated with oral antibiotics.

Particularly among people with diabetes or a weakened immune system, swimmer's ear may lead to infection of the bones and cartilage at the base of the skull (necrotizing otitis externa). This is often accompanied by increasingly severe pain. Such a complication can be life-threatening and usually requires prolonged antibiotic therapy under the care of a team of specialists.

Benign tumors

Benign tumors, or exostoses may develop in the ear canal, caused by an overgrowth of bone. The tumors can grow large enough to block the ear canal and trap wax and water. Ear infection also may develop.

This condition is known as surfer's ear because it develops in so many individuals who participate in surfing. That's because the growths are associated with prolonged exposure to water and wind. Furthermore, the colder the water temperature, the higher the risk — in general, cold-water surfers are more likely to develop exostoses than are warm-water surfers.

The exostoses are slow growing and often present no problem. Should they block the ear canal, they can be surgically removed. This is an outpatient procedure, but recovery may require several weeks, during which time the ear canal is kept dry. Antibiotics can take care of infection, although treatment in a partially blocked canal is more difficult than in an open canal.

Eardrum problems

Your eardrum (tympanic membrane) is a resilient structure but subject to constant strain. Two common problems are rupture of the eardrum membrane and barotrauma. Both conditions prevent the eardrum from vibrating properly, which disrupts the relay of sound waves into the middle ear. This results in mild to moderate hearing loss, which is usually temporary.

Ruptured eardrum

Your eardrum is a thin, elastic membrane that plays the crucial role of gatekeeper for the sound waves traveling from your outer ear to your middle ear. Occasionally, the eardrum may be torn or perforated as a result of an ear infection or from ear trauma.

Ear infection. Fluid buildup in the middle ear caused by infection can exert strong pressure on the eardrum, forcing it to rupture. Pain associated with the buildup usually goes away once the eardrum has ruptured — because fluid draining out of the ear relieves the pressure. But chronic ear infections can gradually wear down the eardrum membrane, even if there is no pressure buildup, causing a tear.

Trauma to the ear. The eardrum can be ruptured by a sharp blow to the head or by a sudden increase in outside air pressure, such as from an explosion, slap across the ear or diving accident. The eardrum also can be punctured if you push an object such as a cotton swab or paper clip into the ear canal.

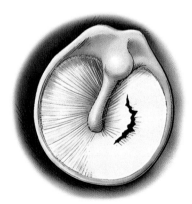

Ruptured eardrum
Although a ruptured eardrum usually will heal itself, the risk of infection and hearing loss still exists. It's important to see your doctor if you think your eardrum may be damaged.

Signs and symptoms of a ruptured eardrum include earache, partial hearing loss, tinnitus (noise such as ringing, buzzing or roaring in your ears) and slight bleeding or discharge from the ear. In some cases the ossicles in the middle ear may be damaged, resulting in more severe hearing loss.

Treatment. Often, a ruptured eardrum heals by itself without complications and with little or no permanent hearing loss. Large ruptures may cause recurring infections.

If you think you may have a ruptured eardrum, contact your doctor immediately. The following self-care tips may ease ear pain and promote healing:
- Take aspirin or other pain relievers, if needed.
- Place a warm — not hot — heating pad over your ear.
- Keep your ear dry.
- Before showering, place a cotton ball coated with petroleum jelly into the ear canal to keep water out.

Your doctor may prescribe an antibiotic to make sure the infection is out of your ear and to help prevent it from recurring. He or she may also place a thin paper patch over your eardrum to seal the opening while it heals. If your eardrum hasn't healed within several months, you may require a surgical procedure to repair the tear.

Barotrauma

Barotrauma (bar-o-TRAW-muh), also called airplane ear, results from a sharp difference between the air pressure in your middle ear and the outside pressure in your environment.

Normally, the eustachian tube, the narrow channel that connects your ear to your nose and upper throat, allows air to flow in and out of your middle ear. This air movement helps equalize pressure on both sides of the eardrum. You may notice clicks or popping sounds in your ears when you swallow or yawn to equalize the pressure.

Barotrauma occurs when you experience a sudden, drastic change in outside air pressure or water pressure, such as a rapid descent during an airplane landing or a rapid ascent during a deep-sea dive.

The rapid change in outside pressure — or restricted airflow in the eustachian tube — can create a situation where air pressure in your middle ear is less than the outside pressure. This imbal-ance causes the air-filled parts of your ear to compress and your eardrum to bow inward (retract). The distortion of your eardrum interferes with the passage of sound waves, so your hearing will be slightly reduced.

Your participation in activities that may involve rapid changes in outside pressure can require you to open your mouth or swallow frequently to equalize the pressure in your ears. Signs and symptoms of barotrauma include pain in one or both ears, slight hearing loss and feeling that both ears are plugged.

A more serious problem occurs if the pressure change is extreme or if your eustachian tube is completely blocked.

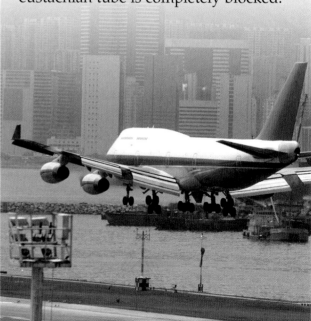

Small blood vessels in your middle ear may rupture, filling your ear with blood and resulting in hearing loss.

Treatment. Although barotrauma may cause discomfort, it doesn't result in permanent hearing loss. The pain usually disappears within a few hours after the pressure has equalized, and your hearing returns to normal.

If you must fly while you have a cold or nose congestion, try a decongestant nasal spray (Afrin, Neo-Synephrine, others) one hour before the flight. This helps keep your eustachian tubes clear. Don't use an oral decongestant if you have a heart condition or blood pressure problems without first obtaining your doctor's approval.

During the flight, suck on candy or chew gum to encourage swallowing. A method used by pilots is to pinch the nostrils shut, inhale and swallow, or to close the nostrils and try to blow air out the ears. The pop in your ears is a sign that air has gone through the eustachian tube to your middle ear.

If symptoms persist, consult your doctor. If the eustachian tube remains obstructed or unable to perform its function, it may become necessary to make a small incision in your eardrum. This helps equalize air pressure and allows fluid to drain from your middle ear — a procedure known as myringotomy (mir-ing-GOT-o-me).

Middle ear problems

Infections, cysts, tumors and abnormal bone growth can affect your middle ear. These problems cause hearing loss when they disturb the eardrum or the tiny bones in the middle ear: the hammer (malleus), anvil (incus) and stirrup (stapes). Often, normal hearing can be restored with medical or surgical treatment. However, if the problem is left untreated and allowed to expand into the inner ear, permanent hearing loss may result.

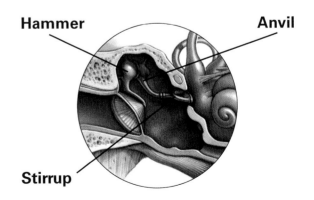

Hammer   Anvil

Stirrup

Middle ear infection

An infection of the middle ear is known as otitis media. The condition is associated with colds and other upper respiratory infections, which can block the eustachian tube. The blocked tube prevents proper ventilation of the ear, causing swelling, inflammation and buildup of fluid in the middle ear.

In addition, bacteria from the nose, mouth or throat may travel through the lining of the eustachian tube and infect the trapped fluid in the middle ear, which causes a thick mucus or pus to form. Infected fluid usually causes ear pain. It may also obstruct proper movement of the eardrum and ossicles, causing conductive hearing loss.

Rarely, pressure from an infection may tear or rupture the eardrum. When this happens, the tear usually heals quickly, without lasting problems. Acute otitis media is a single, severe episode that typically lasts no more than two weeks.

The signs and symptoms of otitis media include:
- Severe pain or pressure in the ear
- Fever above 100.4 degrees Fahrenheit

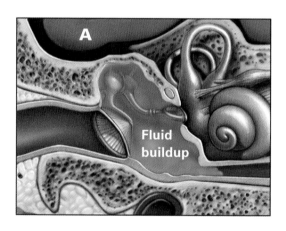 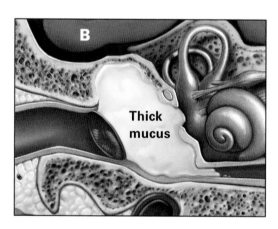

Middle ear infection

(A) Otitis media may occur when the eustachian tube becomes blocked due to a cold or other respiratory infection. Fluid may build up in the normally air-filled middle ear.

(B) Bacteria from the nose and throat may infect the trapped fluid, forming a thick mucus or pus that obstructs movement of the eardrum and ossicles.

- Disrupted sleep
- Sensation of a plugged ear

Other signs and symptoms associated with otitis media are dizziness, imbalance, nausea, vomiting and drainage from the ear.

Although otitis media may occur at any age, it's most common in young children between 4 months and 5 years of age. This is partly due to the shape of a child's eustachian tube, which is shorter and more horizontal than an adult's. A horizontal orientation means fluid is less likely to drain and more likely to accumulate in the ear.

The trapped fluid is an ideal breeding ground for bacteria or viruses that cause infection. At times, the fluid remains trapped, even after the infection is gone. This may cause recurring infections (see "Chronic ear infection").

Treatment. The pain, fever or drainage that's often associated with a middle ear infection will likely cause you to see a doctor. An examination of your ear may reveal a red, bulging or indented eardrum. Tympanometry, which measures movement of the eardrum, may indicate reduced pressure in the middle ear or diminished mobility of the eardrum membrane. Your doctor may take a sample of the draining fluid to identify the organism that's causing the infection.

Studies have found that most ear infections heal on their own without medical treatment. You and your doctor may decide to hold off on using antibiotics and follow a course of watchful waiting. If fluid in the ear isn't infected or if the infection is viral rather than bacterial, the antibiotics provide no benefits — and research shows that viruses cause most ear infections.

To ease ear pain, use over-the-counter pain relievers such as ibuprofen (Advil, Motrin, others) or acetaminophen (Tylenol, others). Applying a cold pack or cold wet washcloth to the outer ear for 20 minutes can help while the medicine takes effect. If you prefer, a warm compress may be used instead of a cold pack. Taking an antihistamine or decongestant may improve nasal breathing and help increase airflow through the eustachian tube.

In follow-up visits, you and your doctor will check to see if the ear infection gets better or worse and to watch for signs of more severe illness. These signs include severe pain, high fever, stiff neck, dehydration, difficulty breathing and extreme irritability.

If the acute symptoms last more than 48 to 72 hours, an antibiotic may be prescribed to fight the infection. Unless the exact organism causing the infection is identified, your doctor will probably prescribe an antibiotic that's effective against a range of bacteria. If the infection doesn't respond to one kind of antibiotic, your doctor may prescribe a different one.

After the infection is gone, fluid in the middle ear usually disappears within three to 12 weeks. Once you begin taking antibiotics, it's important to complete the full prescription, even if your symptoms improve. This ensures that all of the bacteria are killed.

Chronic ear infection

Chronic otitis media is a recurring or persistent middle ear infection. Sometimes, a low-level infection con-

Key points

Keep in mind the following points regarding acute ear infections:
- Ear pain and possible ear infections do not typically require urgent medical attention.
- Most ear infections are not serious and will heal on their own without the use of antibiotics.
- Ear pain can be successfully controlled with pain relievers and other pain management strategies.
- Physicians most often recommend antibiotics for ear infections when ear pain lasts more than 48 to 72 hours, or if you show signs of a more severe illness.
- If you're beginning to experience signs or symptoms of a more severe illness, seek immediate medical care.

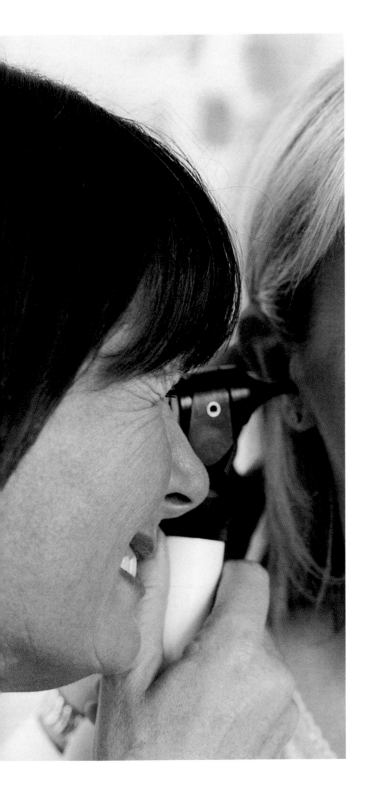

tinues even after you've been treated for acute otitis media. Other times, the acute infection clears up but the ear is left more vulnerable to future infections. Persistent inflammation of the adenoid tissue behind your nasal passages may also cause swelling and block the eustachian tube.

The signs and symptoms of chronic ear infection may appear milder than those of acute infection — in fact, a chronic condition may not be noticed until after the infection is established. But a chronic infection can be more harmful than an acute one because it can cause permanent ear damage and hearing loss.

When the eustachian tube is frequently blocked, tissues of the middle ear gradually begin to thicken and inflame. Mucus trapped in the middle ear also thickens. A vacuum created in the middle ear by the blocked tube can, over time, deform or rupture the eardrum.

As these changes come about, the structures of the middle and inner ear begin to deteriorate, causing permanent damage and hearing impairment. Infection can also spread to the bone behind the ear — a projection of bone called the mastoid process — and even to the brain.

Seek medical attention if pus is seeping from your ear canal, if your ear continually hurts, or you experience hearing loss. Your doctor can refer you to an audiologist to determine the type and severity of hearing loss.

The doctor may also try to identify the source of infection. A computerized tomography (CT) scan may be taken to check if infection has spread to the mastoid process.

Treatment. Your doctor may prescribe antihistamines or decongestants if nasal congestion from a cold or allergy is contributing to the infection. This will help open the eustachian tube, improve nasal breathing and increase airflow to and from the middle ear.

If you have had multiple or frequent ear infections — usually three or more ear infections in a six-month period or four infections within 12 months — your doctor may suggest a low-dose antibiotic over several weeks strictly as a preventive measure. Preventive antibiotics won't help clear fluid from the middle ear, but they may prevent bacterial growth.

Unfortunately, even while taking antibiotics, an ear infection can still occur. Because widespread, prolonged use of antibiotics has contributed to the growth of drug-resistant bacteria, doctors don't agree on whether antibiotics should be used preventively.

If the middle ear remains fluid-filled for more than three months and the eardrum is not ruptured, a small surgical incision in your eardrum may be necessary to relieve pressure and help drain fluid. Hearing often improves immediately following the procedure.

Typically, it takes less than 10 minutes to make the tiny incision, suction out the fluid, and insert a metal or plastic tube into the hole. This ventilation tube keeps the drainage pathway open. If not for the tube, the incision usually heals in about a week — sometimes before all of the fluid has drained out.

If significant damage has occurred to the eardrum and ossicles, surgery may be needed to remove infected tissue and repair these structures. This procedure is known as tympanomastoidectomy (tim-puh-no-mas-toid-EK-tuh-me).

The entire procedure may be done all at once, or an initial surgery may be undertaken only to eliminate the infection. Later surgery is performed to reconstruct the middle ear structures. Chronic ear infections often require multiple surgeries.

Cholesteatoma

Cholesteatoma (ko-luh-ste-uh-TO-muh) is a benign tumor commonly found in the middle ear or the mastoid process. It can occur when skin from the ear canal grows into the middle ear through a hole or tear in the eardrum. It may also happen when a blocked eustachian tube creates a vacuum in the middle ear, bending your eardrum inward to form a pocket. Old skin cells that are caught in the eardrum pocket develop into a cyst-like cholesteatoma.

Occasionally during fetal development, skin cells become trapped behind the eardrum so that a baby is born with congenital cholesteatoma. Unlike the adult form, this type of cholesteatoma may grow quickly.

Signs and symptoms of cholesteatoma include pus drainage from your ear, hearing loss, ear pain or numbness, headache, dizziness, and weakness of the facial muscles.

The degree of hearing loss will depend on the size and location of the tumor.

Frequently, it impedes the function of the ossicles, causing significant conductive hearing loss.

A cholesteatoma isn't cancerous and won't spread to other locations. If left untreated, it can erode bony structures of the middle ear and the mastoid process. It may also affect the cochlea and vestibular labyrinth of the inner ear — resulting in permanent hearing loss and problems with balance. A cholesteatoma may damage the facial nerve and, rarely, cause meningitis, an infection of the central nervous system.

Treatment. A cholesteatoma can only be treated surgically. A large or more advanced cholesteatoma may require a series of operations to correct damage to the bones of your middle ear and possibly to rebuild them. If all of the tumor isn't removed, it will grow back, possibly requiring later surgery.

In severe cases when the cholesteatoma is large or located in an area of the ear that's difficult to access, the surgeon may perform a mastoidectomy (mas-toid-EK-tuh-me) to remove damaged portions of the mastoid bone. This leaves a cavity that must be cleaned out periodically, but doesn't restore damaged bones or lost hearing.

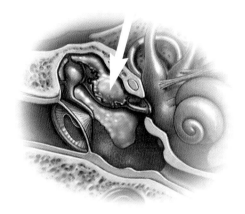

Cholesteatoma

The untreated tumor (see arrow) has eroded bones in the middle ear and ruptured the eardrum. Surgical removal of the tumor may require patching the eardrum and replacing the ossicles with a prosthesis.

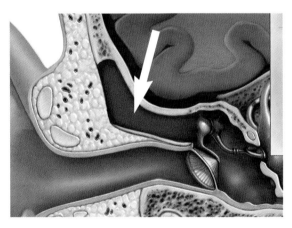

Mastoidectomy

Damaged bone in the mastoid caused by a cholesteatoma has been removed to stop the disease process (see arrow).

Subsequent surgery may be undertaken to reconstruct the ossicular chain in the middle ear, if it has been damaged.

Other cysts and tumors

Abnormal growths may develop in the middle ear and surrounding tissues, such as the temporal bone of the skull — although these types of growths are less common.

Most middle ear tumors are noncancerous (benign), although some, such as squamous cell carcinoma, are cancerous (malignant) and capable of spreading to other parts of the body. Benign tumors usually grow slowly, whereas malignant tumors tend to grow at a faster rate.

The sensation of a plugged ear may indicate a tumor. Other warning signs include hearing loss, tinnitus (noise such as ringing, buzzing or roaring in your ears), drainage from the ear, facial paralysis, dizziness and loss of balance.

Consult your doctor if you experience any of these symptoms. A CT or MRI scan can help determine if a tumor is present. Your doctor may take sample tissue from the tumor (biopsy) to determine whether it's malignant.

The more common tumors include:

Glomus tympanicum and glomus jugulare. Both types of tumor are masses of cells that interfere with the function of the ossicles. Often a glomus tumor will cause a pulsing sound in your ear that accompanies each heartbeat. Most glomus tumors are benign, although rarely they can spread to the lymph nodes in your neck and become a more serious problem.

Squamous cell carcinoma. Malignant tumors of the ear are rare, but of those which occur, squamous cell carcinoma (SKWAY-mus sel kahr-sih-NO-muh) is the most common. This type of tumor develops in the skin cells of your outer ear and ear canal and spreads into your middle ear and mastoid.

Though what causes the tumor is unclear, it has been associated with chronic inflammation. Ear pain, periodic draining of fluid from the ear and extended periods of bleeding from the ear are signs and symptoms of squamous cell carcinoma. This cancer is usually fatal if left untreated.

Tumors of the ear may be treated with surgery, radiation or both. Sometimes, the tumors may also be monitored with watchful waiting, especially in older adults. With this approach, regular MRI or CT scans are taken to check the tumor for growth.

When surgery is performed, it's a delicate, complex procedure and may involve removing some or all parts of the ear, depending on the nature and size of the tumor. This can result in permanent loss of hearing, as well as loss of function in the nerves leading to your face and shoulder.

Radiation therapy may be used as a primary treatment or in combination with surgery to improve the chances of controlling the tumor. With any malignant tumor, treatment must be prompt and aggressive. Radiation therapy is often used after surgery to destroy all remaining cancerous cells.

Otosclerosis

Otosclerosis (o-to-skluh-RO-sis) develops when an abnormal growth of spongy bone forms at the entrance to the inner ear (oval window). Due to this growth, the stirrup, one of the tiny bones in the middle ear, becomes fixed to the oval window, losing its ability to vibrate. The immobile stirrup disrupts the sound pathway.

For some people with otosclerosis, hearing loss can be profound, especially when tissue in the cochlea of the inner ear also becomes involved. Other signs and symptoms of otosclerosis include dizziness, balance problems and tinnitus.

Otosclerosis is a frequent cause of conductive hearing loss in young adults. It's twice as common in women as in men and affects whites more often than individuals of other races. Signs and symptoms of the condition usually appear between the ages of 15 and 35. The disease develops gradually and can affect one or both ears.

An increasing body of evidence suggests that genetic defects may predispose a person to the disease — from among all the individuals who have otosclerosis, approximately half of this population will have a family history of the disease.

Treatment. Because otosclerosis typically results in a mild to moderate hearing loss and doesn't progress far beyond that, hearing aids can successfully overcome most hearing loss due to the condition.

Another treatment option is surgery through the ear canal to replace the fixed stirrup with a tiny wire or prosthesis. This procedure is known as a stapedotomy (stay-puh-DOT-uh-mee). The prosthesis allows sound vibrations to again pass from the eardrum to the

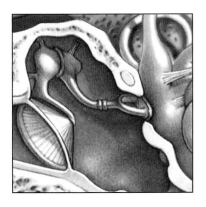 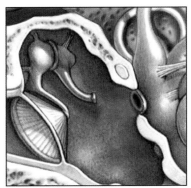 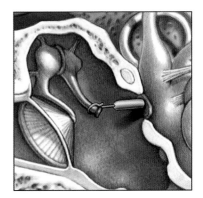

Stapedotomy

With this procedure, a malfunctioning stirrup (stapes) is partly or completely removed and replaced with a tiny wire or prosthesis that resumes the sound pathway to the inner ear.

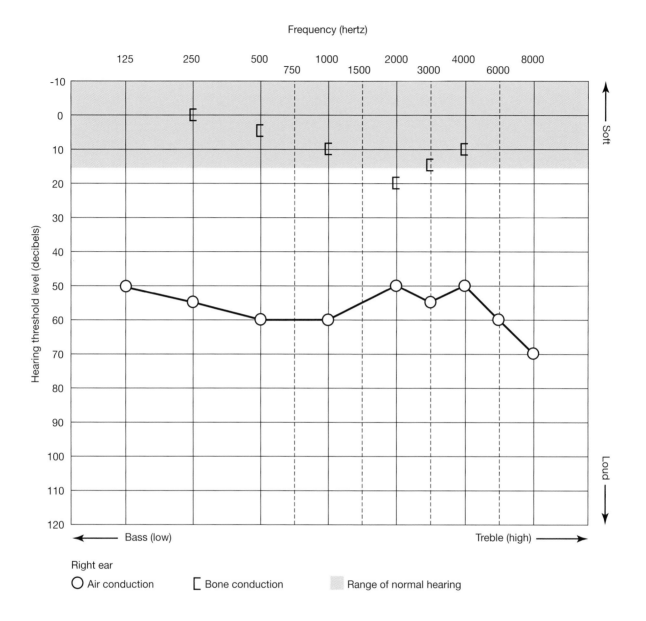

Frequency (hertz)

Otosclerosis

A typical audiogram of hearing loss due to otosclerosis in the right ear. Because the stirrup can no longer vibrate and transmit sound waves to the inner ear, air conduction for all frequencies is far below what is generally considered normal. Bone conduction remains good.

inner ear. Hearing improvement is usually permanent, although it may not be noticeable until about three to six weeks after surgery.

In rare cases, a person undergoing the procedure loses all hearing in the ear. The prosthesis may eventually become displaced, a growth of spongy bone may recur over the oval window, or the anvil (incus), to which the prosthesis is attached, may erode. If the disease progresses after surgery, the function of the prosthesis may be reduced.

If you have otosclerosis, you may be told to take tablets of sodium fluoride, but the value of this treatment is controversial. A rationale for this treatment is that fluoride may help harden the spongy bone, preventing progressive changes in the inner ear and the resulting hearing loss.

Ossicular chain disruption

A traumatic head injury can result in the displacement or breaking (fracture) of the small bones of the middle ear. These bones — the hammer, anvil and stirrup — are referred to collectively as the ossicular chain.

The most common site of displacement from a trauma is at the joint where the anvil connects to the stirrup. Often, the anvil itself is partially broken. The disruption of the ossicular chain causes a breakdown in the sound pathway from the eardrum to the inner ear, resulting in significant hearing loss.

Treatment. Obviously, a complete medical examination should follow any serious head trauma. Tests can help determine the nature of any hearing loss and the degree of its severity. If you still have hearing loss six months after the trauma, your doctor may propose surgery or recommend that you talk to an audiologist about a hearing aid to remedy the loss.

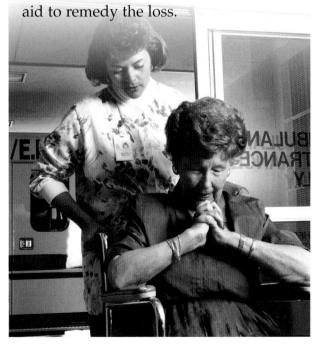

Surgery involves a procedure called ossiculoplasty (os-IH-ku-lo-plas-te), which attempts to rebuild the displaced ossicles or to replace them either with a prosthesis or with small pieces of bone or cartilage. Because the ossicles are so small, the operation is a delicate one, and you may not recover all of your hearing.

If head trauma has damaged the cochlea, resulting in sensorineural hearing loss, a hearing aid may be your best option, as surgery can't be used to correct cochlear damage.

Although complications are rare, some risks that accompany all types of ear surgery are:
- Total deafness in the affected ear
- Tinnitus
- Dizziness and loss of balance
- Damage to the facial nerve resulting in changes to your sense of taste or facial paralysis on the affected side

Your ear doctor will discuss such risks with you before any decision is made regarding surgery.

Chapter 4

Problems of the inner ear

The word *sensorineural* refers to the response of your nerve cells to stimuli from the external environment and from the internal functions of your body. With regard to hearing, the term is associated with the cochlea — the primary structure of the inner ear — and the auditory nerve.

The organ of Corti, located inside the cochlea, contains rows of ultrasensitive receptors known as hair cells, which respond to incoming auditory stimuli. These hair cells convert sound waves into electrical impulses that are carried by the auditory nerve to centers in the brain (see page 18).

Sensorineural (sen-suh-re-NOOR-ul) hearing loss involves damage to the cochlea, the auditory nerve or both. For example, when hair cells in the organ of Corti are damaged due to trauma or simply to the wear and tear of age, the electrical impulses aren't transmitted as efficiently, resulting in hearing loss.

A common form of sensorineural hearing loss is presbycusis (pres-bih-KU-sis). As you get older, the hair cells gradually wear out, causing you to lose some sensitivity to sound. Some adults lose very little hearing as they age, while others lose considerably more due to hair cell loss.

How much hearing loss you experience depends on various genetic and environmental factors, including:

- **Cumulative noise.** A lifetime of hearing the sounds of power tools, machinery, appliances and motor vehicles can gradually affect your ability to hear.
- **Sudden intense noise.** A single loud report from a nearby explosion or gunshot is another cause of sensorineural hearing loss.
- **Medications.** Certain drugs that are harmful to hearing are referred to as ototoxic (oh-toh-TOK-sik).

Other causes of sensorineural hearing loss may be disease, physical trauma and genetic disorders.

Typically, sensorineural damage is permanent and irreversible. But with the use of hearing aids and other assistive devices and techniques, it's possible to communicate effectively despite a sensorineural hearing impairment.

Presbycusis

Presbycusis refers to age-related hearing loss. It's known that hearing tends to decrease as people age. Around 30 percent of Americans who are age 65 and older have hearing loss, whereas only about 3 percent of those under 45 have hearing loss, according to a survey conducted for the Centers for Disease Control and Prevention and the National Center for Health Statistics.

There's a lot of variation in how people age, but in general you can expect the physical and mental changes to cause your senses to become a little less sharp and for sensory details to be a little harder to distinguish. In your ears, for example, you may lose hair cells in the cochlea — probably the most common cause of sensorineural hearing loss. In addition, your brain may not be as quick to interpret incoming signals from the auditory nerve into recognizable sounds.

At first, you may notice that you're losing your sensitivity to sounds that have a high frequency (pitch). That's because the initial damage to hair cells often occurs where high-frequency sounds are processed. When this happens, you may be unable to hear or distinguish between certain sounds of speech, such as *sss, fff* and *thh*.

At the same time, your ability to hear sounds with a low frequency remains intact. Some sounds, such as a boom-

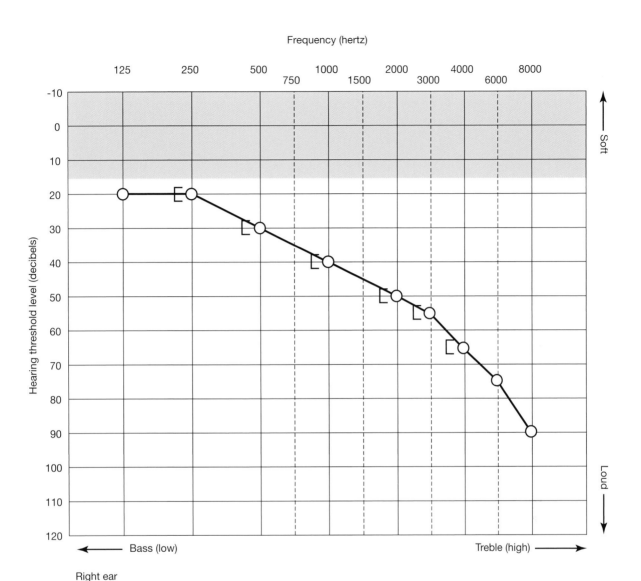

Frequency (hertz)

Bass (low) — Treble (high)

Right ear
○ Air conduction   ⊏ Bone conduction   ▒ Range of normal hearing

Audiogram of presbycusis

Audiogram of the right ear showing a typical pattern of hearing loss due to presbycusis. Often as you age, your sensitivity to low-frequency sounds remains relatively intact but you'll have increasing difficulty hearing high-frequency sounds. Certain high-frequency sounds, such as doorbells or bird songs, may become inaudible.

ing bass instrument or a passing truck, may even seem too loud.

Presbycusis is sometimes accompanied by ringing or buzzing in your ears, which is a condition known as tinnitus (TIN-ih-tus). Presbycusis also makes it hard to hold a conversation in public spaces, such as a busy store or restaurant, where there's often commotion and background noise.

Not being able to hear everything spoken in a conversation is the equivalent of reading a book from which random pages have been removed or having to recognize a song based on the throbbing bass line from a radio at your neighbor's house. It's usually a frustrating, if not annoying, experience.

Presbycusis tends to run in families, which suggests that genetics are involved. Its onset may be earlier in some families than in others.

Just as you adjust to other changes that may accompany aging, such as vision loss and high blood pressure, you can also compensate for presbycusis. In particular, hearing aids can make high-frequency sounds audible without amplifying the low-frequency sounds that you already hear.

Noise-induced hearing loss

Every day we're surrounded by noise — the bustle of traffic, the hums and grinds of machinery, people conversing, music and chatter from the radio, airplanes flying overhead.

Typically we think nothing of these familiar sounds. Most of the time they aren't loud enough to interfere in our routines or hurt our ears. But sometimes a noise is too loud for our ears, and some sounds may cause permanent damage.

A single explosion of noise and prolonged exposure to loud noise are two ways that noise can damage hearing:

- **Single explosion of noise.** Sudden unprotected exposure to a sound measuring 140 dB or above, such as a rifle gunshot or firecracker blast, can cause immediate hearing loss. The sounds of artillery and explosions are more dangerous. In fact, noise-induced hearing loss is a common injury in the military.
- **Prolonged exposure to loud noise.** Long-term exposure to noise levels above 85 dB can damage your hear-

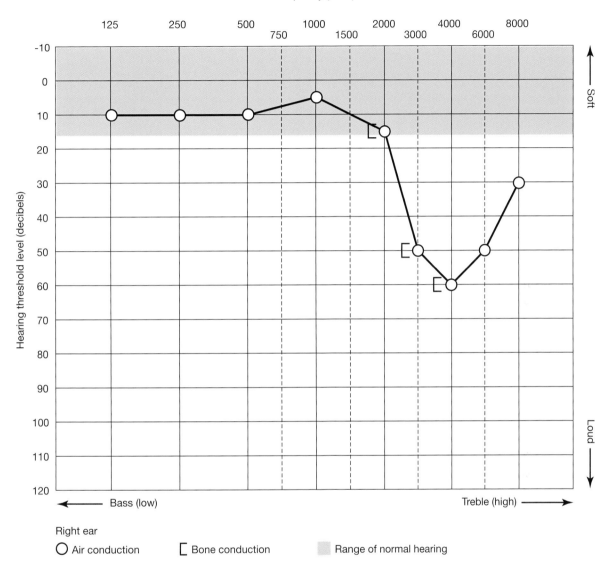

Frequency (hertz)

Right ear
O Air conduction   E Bone conduction   Range of normal hearing

Audiogram of noise-induced hearing loss

Audiogram of the right ear showing a typical pattern of hearing loss due to noise. Hearing sounds at low frequencies may remain in the normal range, while the ability to hear high frequencies takes a characteristic dip, greatest at 4,000 hertz.

Hold down the noise

Most of us are aware of the dangers of work-related noise. But we easily overlook the racket at home. Here are steps you can take to hold down the noise level around your house:

- Turn down the volume on your television or stereo.
- Wear snug-fitting headphones that block background noise on portable music players so that you don't have to turn up the volume so much.
- Choose quieter appliances.
- Place pads under noisy appliances.
- Don't run multiple appliances at the same time.
- Install carpeting to absorb sound.
- Seal windows and doors to block the noise of traffic.
- Wear earplugs or earmuffs when using power equipment.
- Rest your ears. Alternate noisy activities with quiet ones.

Hearing loss that results from many recreational activities is becoming more common. Don't forget to wear ear protectors when riding a snowmobile or motorcycle, practicing at the rifle range, or listening to extremely loud music.

ing. This may happen at work or during recreational activities. Noise sources include power tools, lawn equipment, tractors, motorcycles and snowmobiles, and sound equipment such as portable music players set to high volume.

Noise-induced hearing loss can occur in one or both ears. You may start noticing that familiar sounds seem muffled or distorted, accompanied by the ringing or buzzing in your ears known as tinnitus — which may or may not subside.

Approximate sound levels of noise

Sound level (decibels)	Noise
30	Whisper
40	Refrigerator hum
60	Normal conversation
70	Washing machine
85	Heavy city traffic
95	Motorcycle, power lawn mower
100	Snowmobile, hand drill, blow dryer
110	Chain saw, rock concert
120	Ambulance siren
140	Jet engine at takeoff
165	12-gauge shotgun blast
180	Rocket launch

Adapted from National Institute on Deafness and Other Communication Disorders, 2006, and American Tinnitus Association, 2007

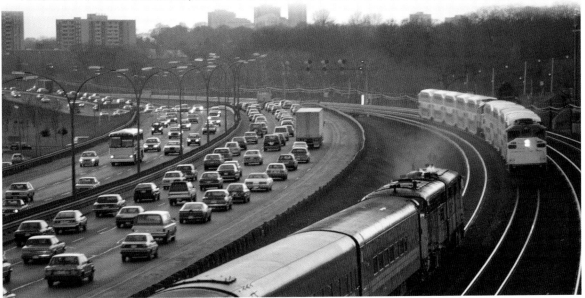

Portable music players

The greatly improved sound quality, small size and convenience of portable music players has translated into more time listening to music. Unfortunately, many users listen for too long at too high a volume. This can cause noise-induced hearing loss, which may not be noticeable until significant damage has occurred.

Portable music players typically produce sound levels ranging between 60 dB and 120 dB. Listening to sounds of 80 dB or less isn't likely to cause damage. Keeping the volume at a level where you can still comfortably carry on a conversation means you won't need to limit the amount of time that you listen. Using earphones that sit over your ear, rather than sit in the ear, may help block background noise, allowing you to listen at lower decibel levels.

While you can't measure the decibel level of your music, there are simple ways to tell if the volume is set too high:
- The volume on your device is set higher than 60 percent of the maximum
- You can't hear conversations going on around you
- People near you can hear your music
- You find yourself shouting when you talk to people nearby

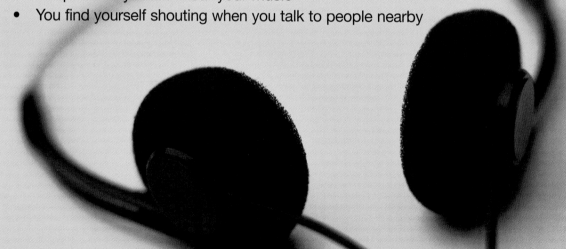

Following sudden exposure to loud noise, you may experience these symptoms immediately. With prolonged exposure, the hearing loss may be so gradual that you're not aware of a problem until you have a hearing test.

If your hearing loss is temporary, it's called a temporary threshold shift. With this condition, normal hearing usually returns within 16 hours of being exposed to noise. But sometimes, hearing loss from your exposure to loud noise may be permanent.

Although noise-induced hearing loss usually can't be restored, there are ways in which it can be prevented:
- Avoid exposure to the loud noise
- Move farther away from its source
- Wear hearing protectors — earmuffs or earplugs — when involved in loud activities.

So how loud is too loud? Here's a good rule of thumb: If you have to shout in order to be heard by someone an arm's length away, you're being exposed to too much noise.

Hearing protectors are effective when they can be worn for the entire time that you're exposed to loud noise. Earplugs are small inserts that fit inside the ear canal. Earmuffs fit over the entire outer ear. They can reduce the noise by about 15 to 30 decibels. When earplugs and earmuffs are worn together, they offer an additional reduction of 5 dB — which is important when noise levels are high.

Whatever type of ear protection you use, make sure it's clean and it fits correctly. Earplugs should maintain an airtight seal in your ear. Earmuffs must contact the skin entirely around your ear. Devices that meet federal standards are available at drugstores, hardware stores and sporting goods stores.

In companies that operate at noise levels averaging 85 dB over an eight-hour day, employers are required to have a hearing conservation program, which includes conventional noise measurements, the provision of hearing protectors to employees, an annual hearing test to screen employees, as well as education and training sessions.

See Chapter 2 for information on screening for hearing loss. If testing reveals significant loss in an employee, he or she is required to wear hearing protectors. If noise levels reach 90 dB or above, everyone is required by law to wear hearing protectors.

Sudden deafness

Sometimes hearing can be lost all at once or within only a few days. This condition is known as sudden sensorineural hearing loss (SSNHL).

SSNHL is almost always confined to one ear. You may notice a popping sound when it happens, or you may detect it when you first wake up or try to use the impaired ear. Dizziness or tinnitus also may develop. About 4,000 cases of sudden deafness occur every year in the United States.

Sudden deafness is an urgent medical concern. If you notice the symptoms, contact your doctor immediately. You'll be checked to determine the extent of hearing loss. And the less hearing loss that has occurred, the more likely that you'll return to normal hearing within a few weeks. Although many individuals with SSNHL regain their former hearing, some may have no recovery or else regain only partial hearing in the affected ear.

Pinpointing the cause of SSNHL can be a difficult task. If your hearing returns quickly, you may not need medical treatment. If the cause is known, taking care of the underlying problem may resolve the hearing loss. When the cause isn't obvious, your doctor may consider several possible suspects, including:

- Viral inner ear infection
- Abrupt disruption of blood flow to the cochlea
- Membrane tear within the cochlea
- Acoustic neuroma

Most of the time the cause is unknown. Your doctor may prescribe a corticosteroid such as prednisone or dexamethasone to reduce the inflammation. Sometimes, the corticosteroid is injected directly into the middle ear through the eardrum, which allows for a higher concentration of the drug to enter the inner ear. The doctor may also prescribe an antiviral medication such as famciclovir (Famvir).

Other causes of hearing loss

Factors other than aging and noise exposure may damage the inner ear and auditory nerve. The sensorineural hearing loss that results may be sudden or may worsen gradually.

Viral infections

Before widespread practice of childhood immunization, the viruses responsible for several illnesses were also major causes of hearing loss. The measles virus usually attacks cells lining the lungs and the back of the throat. The mumps typically affects one of the salivary glands between the ear and the jaw. Either infection may spread to your inner ear and destroy hair cells in the cochlea.

Hearing loss from these illnesses is now rare in the United States because they can be prevented with a vaccine. Children routinely get this shot at ages 12 to 15 months and again at 3 to 6 years. You also gain immunity if you've previously had a measles or mumps infection.

Viruses may also travel through your bloodstream to the cochlea, leading to hearing loss. These viral illnesses include influenza, chickenpox and mononucleosis.

If you're not sure whether you've been immunized or you need a vaccination before traveling to a place where the illnesses are still prevalent, talk to your doctor about the vaccine.

Head trauma

A blow to the head can sometimes cause hearing impairment, especially if the part of the skull containing your ear (temporal bone) is fractured. Such a fracture may damage the delicate structure of the cochlea or your auditory nerve. Damage to the nerve interferes with communication to the brain. Occasionally, hearing loss isn't apparent until some time after the trauma.

Normally, your brain rests inside your skull protected by a cushion of spinal fluid. A sharp blow to the head will cause your brain to shift, which can tear blood vessels, pull nerve fibers and bruise tissue. Pressure waves from the blow can disrupt structures in the cochlea (cochlear concussion) and cause sensorineural hearing loss.

If you've experienced a cochlear concussion, your hearing may improve over a six-month period. Another result of head trauma may be bleeding into the cochlear fluids, which also can result in hearing loss.

Trauma to your head may sometimes rupture the membrane covering the oval window or the round window — two openings between the middle ear

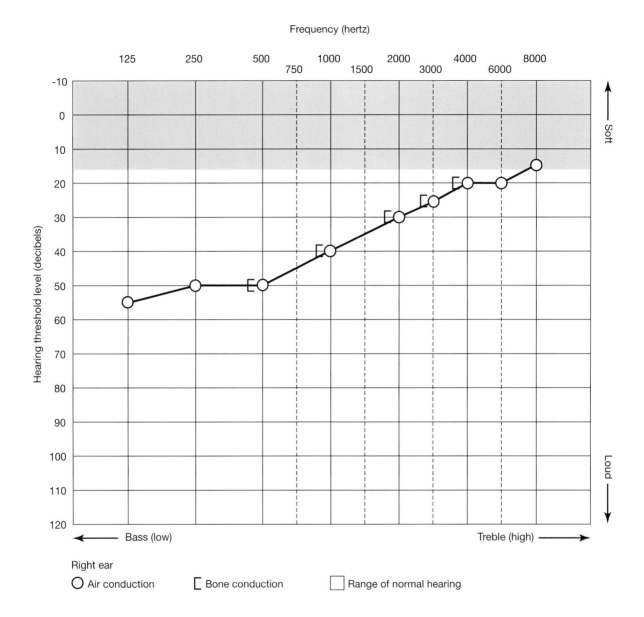

Audiogram of Meniere's disease

Audiogram of the right ear showing how Meniere's disease typically affects hearing. During attacks, sounds at lower and middle frequencies are more difficult to hear than sounds at higher frequencies.

and inner ear. This condition is known as perilymph fistula. The rupture allows fluid to leak into the middle ear, causing hearing impairment. If hearing loss or dizziness persists, exploratory surgery may be recommended.

Meniere's disease

Meniere's (men-e-AYRZ) disease is characterized by periodic attacks when you experience the sensation of spinning or rotating (vertigo), hearing loss, tinnitus, and the feeling of a plugged ear. One attack may last anywhere from 20 minutes to several hours.

The attacks are unpredictable and can occur as often as several times a week or as infrequently as once a year. Typically, dizziness is the worst symptom and may cause nausea. Between attacks you may not feel any symptoms at all. Although hearing comes and goes with the attacks, it may gradually worsen. Meniere's disease usually affects only one ear.

No one knows what causes Meniere's disease, but scientists associate the signs and symptoms with fluctuations in the fluid volume of the inner ear. Excess fluid increases pressure on the membranes of the inner ear, which

may distort and occasionally rupture them. This development affects your hearing and sense of balance.

Treating Meniere's disease usually involves taking medications to manage the symptoms of dizziness and nausea, limiting your intake of caffeine, alcohol and chocolate, and eating a low-salt diet. Limiting salt intake may help decrease fluid levels in your body — including your inner ear — and possibly decrease the frequency of attacks.

Your doctor may also prescribe a diuretic, antihistamine or migraine medication to help reduce fluid retention. Medications such as corticosteroids, which reduce inflammation, or the antibiotic gentamicin, which reduces vestibular activity, may be injected into the middle ear to reduce or eliminate attacks.

If dizziness is severe, inner ear surgery may be an option. For more information on surgery of this kind, see the brief summary on page 222.

Labyrinthitis

Labyrinthitis (lab-uh-rin-THI-tis) is an inflammation that can affect both the cochlea, which is vital to hearing, and the vestibular labyrinth, which plays a role in balance and eye movement. If the inflammation affects only the vestibular labyrinth, it's known as vestibular neuronitis.

The inflammation often follows a bacterial ear infection or a viral upper respiratory illness. Bacterial meningitis can cause severe to profound hearing loss. Vaccinations against the pneumococcal and meningococcal organisms responsible for this infection are now recommended for children and adults. Labyrinthitis may also occur after a blow to the head, or it may occur with no associated illness or trauma.

Signs and symptoms of labyrinthitis include dizziness, hearing loss, tinnitus, nausea, vomiting and involuntary movements of your eyes. You may lose all of your hearing in the affected ear.

To minimize dizziness, it's helpful to frequently sit still and avoid sudden changes of position. Most of the time, the inflammation goes away on its own after a few weeks.

If the underlying problem is bacterial, your doctor may prescribe antibiotics. Drugs to relieve dizziness and nausea may also be recommended.

If the dizziness persists, physical or occupational therapy may be recommended. Many individuals recover completely from labyrinthitis, but some continue to experience problems with balance and hearing loss.

Acoustic neuroma

An acoustic neuroma is a slow-growing, benign tumor on the auditory and vestibular nerves. The tumor results from an uncontrolled growth of Schwann cells covering the nerves. It typically develops within the auditory canal and slowly grows toward the brain cavity. The condition is also known as vestibular schwannoma.

Because an acoustic neuroma affects both the auditory and vestibular nerves, hearing loss and tinnitus in one ear are common signs and symptoms of the disorder. As the tumor grows, it can affect other nerves, causing facial numbness and weakness.

Although an acoustic neuroma is generally slow growing, it can become large enough to push against the brain and interfere with life-sustaining functions. The tumor is usually removed with surgery, but it may also be treated with radiation therapy.

To remove an acoustic neuroma, a surgeon will make a small incision behind or above your ear and remove a segment of your skull in order to get at the tumor. Once the tumor is located and removed, the bony segment is replaced to cover the opening in the skull and protect the brain.

If the tumor can be removed without injuring the auditory nerve, your hearing may be preserved — which is possible if the tumor is small. In general, the larger the tumor, the greater are the chances of your hearing, balance and facial nerves being affected.

A noninvasive treatment to shrink or stabilize small or medium-sized tumors is stereotactic radiosurgery. This closed-skull procedure involves sophisticated imaging that targets several focused radiation beams on a tumor. The separate beams are too weak to harm tissue they pass through — damage occurs only at the spot in the brain where the beams meet.

One of the benefits of this procedure is that the skull isn't opened, eliminating the chances for surgical complications. And recovery time is shorter than with open surgery. A drawback is that the

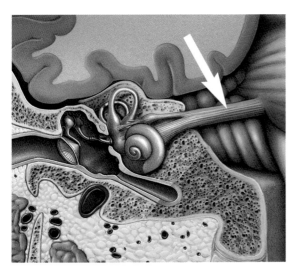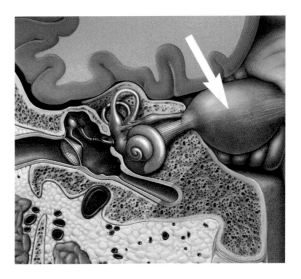

Acoustic neuroma

An acoustic neuroma is a tumor on your auditory nerve. The arrow in the lefthand image shows a normal auditory nerve. The arrow in the righthand image indicates a large tumor that has developed at the base of the bony internal auditory canal.

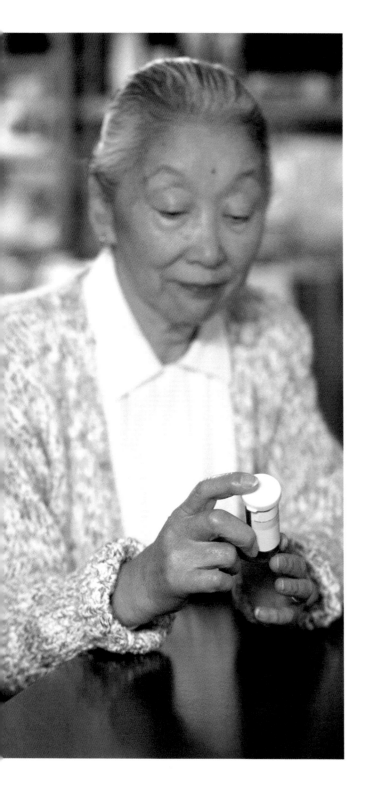

tumor is not removed — although it's hoped that the radiation will stabilize it or shrink its size.

Reaction to medications

The action of certain medications or chemicals can cause hearing loss, tinnitus and balance problems. Medications can also aggravate an existing hearing problem. These medications are considered ototoxic.

The effects of ototoxic medications can range from mild to severe. It generally depends on the dosage strength and on the length of time you take the drugs. Common ototoxic medications are listed on pages 94-95.

Hearing problems caused by some ototoxic drugs will go away after you stop taking the medications. Drugs that are known to cause permanent hearing loss are usually given only when no other option exists for treating a life-threatening disease.

About 200 medications are considered ototoxic. If you and your doctor decide that it's in your best interest to take an ototoxic drug, an audiologist will likely test your hearing before, during and after you take the drug.

While you're taking the ototoxic drug, your physician will closely monitor test results to determine how long you can continue with the regimen or when to alter the dosage.

Signs and symptoms of an ototoxic reaction include:

- Onset of tinnitus
- Worsening of existing tinnitus
- Feeling that one or both ears are plugged
- Loss of hearing or worsening of existing hearing loss
- Dizziness, sometimes accompanied by nausea

Notify your doctor if you have an existing hearing or balance problem or if you experience inner ear problems from certain medications. This may help you avoid unnecessary exposure to ototoxic drugs. If needed, an audiologist can help you plan for a hearing aid and hearing rehabilitation.

Autoimmune inner ear disease

Autoimmune inner ear disease (AIED) occurs when your body's immune system mistakes normal cells in your inner ear for a virus or bacteria and begins attacking them. This produces an inflammatory reaction that can lead to problems with both hearing and balance. AIED is rare, probably accounting for less than 1 percent of all cases of hearing loss.

It's unknown why the immune cells start attacking other normal cells. As with many other disorders, scientists suspect that AIED may have something to do with abnormal genetics.

A characteristic of AIED is hearing loss that progresses rapidly in both ears, occurring over weeks or months. Sometimes, the hearing loss starts in one ear and moves to the other.

Other signs and symptoms include tinnitus, a plugged ear and, in about half the AIED cases, dizziness. Because these signs and symptoms are similar to those of many other ear disorders, diagnosis can be difficult.

In addition, AIED is often associated with other autoimmune disorders of the body, such as:

- Ankylosing spondylitis, a disease that affects your spine
- Sjögren's syndrome, also known as dry eye syndrome
- Cogan's syndrome, which affects your eyes and ears

Ototoxic medications

Listed below are some of the drugs that may cause hearing loss. If you're taking one of these medications, it's important not to stop taking it until you've consulted your doctor.

Class of drugs	Examples	Effects
Salicylates	• Aspirin • Aspirin-containing products	Ototoxicity usually occurs at high doses. Hearing loss is almost always reversible.
Quinine	• Chloroquine (Aralen) • Quinidine • Quinine (Quinamm) • Tonic water	Ototoxicity usually occurs at high doses. Hearing improves when use of the drug is stopped.
Loop diuretics (a specific type of water pill)	• Bumetanide (Bumex) • Ethacrynic acid (Edecrin) • Furosemide (Lasix) • Torsemide (Demadex)	Ototoxicity is temporary. If these drugs are given with an ototoxic antibiotic, risk of permanent damage may increase.

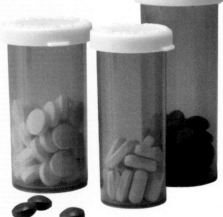
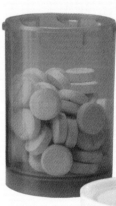

Class of drugs	Examples	Effects
Amino-glycoside antibiotics	• Amikacin (Amikin) • Gentamicin • Neomycin (Mycifradin) • Streptomycin • Tobramycin (Nebcin) • Vancomycin (Vancocin)	Risk of ototoxicity usually increases when the antibiotic is administered directly into the bloodstream, which allows the greatest amount of the drug into the body. Damage may be permanent.
Anti-cancer drugs (anti-neoplastics)	• Carboplatin (Paraplatin) • Cisplatin (Platinol)	Drugs designed to kill cancer cells may also kill inner ear cells. The damage is often permanent and may make you more vulnerable to noise-induced hearing loss.
Environmental chemicals	• Lead • Manganese • n-butyl alcohol • Toluene	Excessive exposure to these chemicals in the workplace may result in permanent hearing loss.

- Ulcerative colitis, which affects your intestinal tract
- Wegener's granulomatosis, which inflames blood vessels
- Rheumatoid arthritis, which inflames your joints
- Scleroderma, which affects your skin and other connective tissues
- Systemic lupus erythematosus (SLE) and Behcet's syndrome, both of which can affect multiple systems in your body

If you have AIED, your doctor may prescribe oral corticosteroids (prednisone, dexamethasone) to reduce the inflammation. Corticosteroids are the most effective treatment for AIED but have side effects that can limit long-term use. In certain cases, steroids may be injected directly into the ear in an attempt to avoid the side effects.

Several treatment options that have been used in the past but are less commonly used today include certain immunosuppressive agents such as methotrexate (Folex, Rheumatrex) that suppress your immune cells, and etanercept (Enbrel), which blocks a protein triggering some of the inflammation. An expensive procedure known as plasmapheresis (plaz-muh-fuh-RE-sis) withdraws blood, mechanically removes the offending antibodies and returns clean blood to your body.

If AIED has caused you to lose much of your hearing in both ears, then you may consider a cochlear implant as a treatment option.

Congenital hearing problems

A congenital problem means the condition exists at birth. These types of hearing problems may be hereditary in nature, but can also develop in the womb or during the birthing process.

Genetic factors may be responsible for more than half of all incidents of congenital hearing loss. A child whose hearing loss is inherited usually has two parents who carry a recessive gene for hearing loss (autosomal recessive hearing loss). This gene isn't expressed in the parents, who have normal hearing, but is expressed in the child who inherits both recessive genes. So far, multiple genes have been identified that cause recessive hearing loss not related to other illnesses.

Often, congenital hearing loss is part of a collection of symptoms (known as a syndrome) caused by a genetic defect.

These conditions include Down syndrome, Usher's syndrome, Treacher Collins syndrome, Crouzon's disease and Alport's syndrome.

Other factors that may cause hearing loss in an infant include:
- Infection in the mother, such as German measles (rubella), cytomegalovirus, herpes or syphilis
- Premature birth
- Lack of oxygen during or shortly after birth
- Blood incompatibilities between mother and child
- Diabetes in the mother
- Fetal alcohol syndrome
- Inner ear malformations such as Mondini malformation

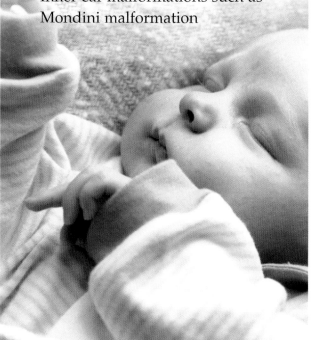

Most newborns will be screened for hearing loss before they leave the hospital. Even with normal results, it's important to continue monitoring your child's hearing, because a hearing impairment that goes unnoticed may significantly interfere with speech and language development. The impairment may be corrected with hearing aids and cochlear implants.

Research on the horizon

The fact that sensorineural damage to the inner ear so often causes severe or profound permanent hearing loss has challenged scientists to come up with new approaches for treatment. They're testing certain drugs that may reduce the effects of noise exposure on the inner ear. They're also studying drugs that may inhibit the effects of aging on your hearing.

Hair cell regeneration

An exciting area of new research involves hair cell regeneration. Hair cells are the delicate sensory receptors of the inner ear, and damage can result in serious hearing problems.

Until recently, scientists believed the inner ear was incapable of producing new hair cells. Then they discovered that birds have a natural ability to generate new hair cells in response to damage. Furthermore, the new cells restored the birds' hearing. This discovery has led researchers to consider how to regenerate lost or damaged hair cells in humans.

Human hair cells might be regenerated using hormone-like substances called growth factors, which regulate cell growth. Researchers are testing various growth factors to identify ones that might cause the hair cells to develop. Their efforts have successfully induced the first stage of hair cell regeneration in the inner ears of mammals such as guinea pigs, rats and mice.

Although progress so far is promising, many challenges remain. Researchers must not only identify the chemical substances that cause regeneration but also find a workable method of delivering these substances to the inner ear.

Gene therapy

Scientists have also made important progress in understanding the relationship between genetics and hearing loss.

They've discovered that many genes can affect hearing and that genetics and environment likely interact to cause hearing loss. For example, an individual may be genetically predisposed to hearing loss caused by specific environmental factors such as noise exposure, drugs or illness.

With this growing body of knowledge, researchers are investigating gene therapy as a way to treat hearing loss. Gene therapy, also called gene transfer, involves replacing a defective gene with a normal gene, with the hope that a cell will accept and use it.

Gene therapy holds great potential for treating hereditary forms of deafness, preventing hair cell damage and stimulating hair cell regeneration. Research is still at an early stage. There's still a long way to go before effective and affordable genetic treatment for hearing impairment is feasible.

Tinnitus

Tinnitus (TIN-ih-tus) is the perception of sound in your ear caused by no apparent external source. The sound is characterized as ringing, buzzing, whistling, chirping, hissing, roaring or clicking, among other descriptions. Some people refer to it as music or the sound of boiling water.

Regardless of how it's described, it's a sound that's not produced in your surroundings. Often the noise seems to originate in your head. In some parts of the country, tinnitus can also be pronounced as tih-NI-tus.

Many people experience brief episodes of tinnitus after being exposed to an extremely loud noise or by taking certain medications. But few people are overly alarmed by such episodes, and the noise usually goes away.

An estimated 50 million adults in the United States experience some degree of a more persistent form of tinnitus. It's usually a benign condition, and most don't find it bothersome.

However, approximately 8 million to 12 million Americans *are* bothered by persistent tinnitus — some more severely than others are. The impact of tinnitus on their lives ranges anywhere from annoying to debilitating. At night the ringing or hissing noise makes it difficult for some of them to fall asleep. Tinnitus also makes it hard for them to focus on their jobs during the day and complete particular tasks.

Frustration with the unexplained sounds can often lead to anxiety, fear and depression. Tinnitus is a symptom associated with many other ear disorders as well as with other diseases, including cardiovascular disease, allergies and anemia.

Unraveling the mystery

Physicians and medical researchers have grappled with a precise definition of tinnitus. It's unclear whether tinnitus is a syndrome — a set of symptoms that accompanies another disorder — or whether it's a disorder in itself.

What mechanisms trigger tinnitus within the ear — which might explain how and why the noise occurs — are unknown. Although descriptions of tinnitus exist as far back as the time of the Pharaohs of ancient Egypt, much about the condition remains a mystery.

Several theories have been proposed regarding the cause of tinnitus. One hypothesis is that it's a phenomenon of the central nervous system, similar to the phantom-like sensations experienced after a limb amputation. A person may feel pain in his or her foot even after the leg has been removed. In similar fashion, the central nervous system is somehow responding to hair cells that have been lost by stimulating electric signals to the brain.

Another theory suggests the disorder is somehow centered in the brain. This evidence is based on positron emission tomography (PET) scans, which reveal the specific parts of the brain that are used to accomplish specific tasks. Careful study of PET imagery of people with the condition suggests that tinnitus sounds stimulate a part of the brain that's different from the parts stimulated by external sounds.

Some researchers speculate that tinnitus arises in the cochlea, specifically from disorganized activity of the hair cells. Others think the cause may lie with the activity of chemicals in the auditory nerve, which carries messages between your inner ear and the brain. Tinnitus may also stem from turbulent blood flow through arteries and veins that lie close to the inner ear.

Evidence also suggests that spontaneous nerve activity may be a culprit. That is, one or more of the auditory

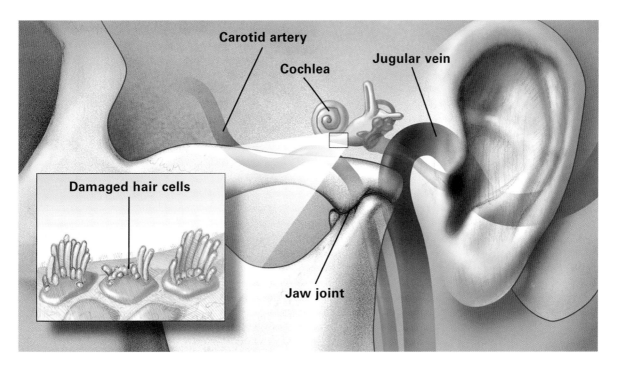

Carotid artery

Cochlea

Jugular vein

Damaged hair cells

Jaw joint

Possible causes of tinnitus

Tinnitus may develop from multiple causes. Some researchers believe that tinnitus results from damage to the hair cells inside your cochlea. Turbulent flow through your blood vessels may produce a sound sensation. Blood vessels such as the carotid artery and the jugular vein lie close to the inner ear. Tinnitus may also result from a misalignment of the jaw joint (temporomandibular joint), which can produce a clicking or grating sound.

information-processing stations in the brain may generate abnormal activity. For some people, physical movement of the body such as teeth clenching or certain neck motions may generate a form of tinnitus.

Regardless of their preferred theory, most scientists agree that multiple causes are probably involved in the development of tinnitus. Unfortunately for those with a condition that's persistent and bothersome, this lack of knowledge has often left them with no recourse but to live with discomfort.

The good news is that tinnitus is generally not a serious or life-threatening medical concern. In a few cases, tinnitus may be caused by an underlying condition that's treatable. More often there's no cure.

But you can learn various ways to manage tinnitus so that its effect on your daily life is minimized. These options often require the assistance of a physician and audiologist along with your active participation.

Types

How people describe tinnitus varies greatly from one person to the next. The only thing they have in common seems to be the existence of an unexplained noise in their head or ears.

To provide a general framework on which to classify tinnitus, some experts have categorized the condition in terms of two broadly defined types: objective and subjective.

Objective tinnitus

Objective tinnitus, sometimes referred to as pulsatile (PUL-suh-tile) tinnitus, is a sound sensation that can be heard by other people as well as by you. The sounds originate within your body, most commonly from turbulent blood flow in your arteries and veins.

If you have atherosclerosis, for example, a buildup of cholesterol and other fatty deposits causes blood vessels to lose elasticity. This restricts the vessels from flexing slightly with each heartbeat. Narrower openings require a more forceful blood flow. Your heart works harder — to the point where your ears can detect each heartbeat. Your doctor may hear the sound with the help of a stethoscope.

High blood pressure, and factors such as stress, alcohol and caffeine that may temporarily increase blood pressure, can make tinnitus more noticeable. Repositioning your head usually can cause the sounds to disappear.

The malformation of small blood vessels (capillaries) connecting your arteries and veins also produces an audible pulse. Other sources of objective tinnitus include muscle spasms, movement of the eustachian tube and spontaneous vibrations of hair cells.

About 4 percent of all the individuals who have tinnitus have the objective type. Treating the underlying vascular disorder, such as atherosclerosis, may help reduce or even eliminate the sounds. That's why it's important to describe the tinnitus to your doctor and receive an accurate diagnosis. Be as specific as you can about the noises you hear and under what circumstances they occur.

Subjective tinnitus

Subjective tinnitus involves sounds that only you detect. Scientists aren't sure what causes these sounds. And in order to study the problem, they must depend on how well people describe what they're hearing.

Hyperacusis

Hyperacusis (hi-pur-uh-KOO-sis) is another condition that's often associated with tinnitus. Hyperacusis involves a heightened aversion to sound. Everyday noise, such as traffic, conversation or telephone rings, seems uncomfortably loud. Like tinnitus, the cause of hyperacusis is unknown.

Hyperacusis may be even more debilitating than is tinnitus. A person with severe hyperacusis may avoid social situations for fear of painful noise exposure (phonophobia), choosing instead to stay in a secluded environment with little or no noise. Although some form of hyperacusis may occur in people with hearing loss, those reporting hyperacusis usually have normal hearing.

Treatment consists of counseling and participating in a program that gradually increases your tolerance of normal sounds. This may involve a white noise generator — an electronic device that generates a persistent hissing sound, similar to what you may hear when a radio is tuned between stations. Initially the device is tuned to barely audible levels and then gradually increased to higher levels for regular periods of time.

In fact, some experts have compared their efforts to study subjective tinnitus to the popular fable of four blind men attempting to describe an elephant by touch. Their speculation may turn out to be quite different from reality.

Still, there's a general consensus that the condition originates within the structures of the inner ear or the auditory centers of the brain.

Although the nature of subjective tinnitus remains unclear, several factors are believed to be capable of triggering the condition or making it worse:

Hearing loss. Exposure to loud noise, even for short term, can damage the hair cells in your cochlea and cause permanent hearing loss. About 90 percent of people with tinnitus have some form of noise-induced hearing loss. It may be that the damage to hair cells also causes the tinnitus.

Some researchers believe that age-related hearing loss may also precipitate tinnitus. As the presbycusis muffles sounds from the outside world, existing tinnitus becomes more noticeable. Other conditions that can reduce hearing, such as impacted earwax or ear infection, also may increase tinnitus.

Medications. Over 200 prescription drugs are associated with tinnitus. Some of these drugs are ototoxic and may permanently injure the ear. Usually such prescriptions are made only when absolutely necessary.

Other drugs can produce tinnitus as a side effect. Always discuss potential side effects of any prescription medication with your doctor. After you begin taking the drug, inform your doctor if your hearing is reduced or you experience tinnitus. Stopping the drug or adjusting the dosage often eliminates the problem. If you already have tinnitus, be sure to tell your doctor.

Jaw disorders. A misaligned joint connecting your jaw and the temporal bone of your skull may cause clicking or grating noises whenever you move your jaw. Some people claim the noises are present even when no jaw movement occurs, but this is debatable. A dentist who specializes in treating this joint may correct the misalignment and eliminate the associated noises.

Other factors. Various conditions or lifestyle factors may cause tinnitus:
- Schwannomas (shwah-NO-muhz), which are benign tumors that grow on auditory nerve fibers

- Serious trauma or injury to the head or neck
- Perilymph fistula, a membrane rupture of the oval window or round window (see page 225)
- Otosclerosis, or a stiffening of the ossicle bones in the middle ear
- Meniere's disease, which causes excess fluid in the inner ear
- Exposure to excessive noise
- Too much sodium in your diet
- Stress, either emotional or physical

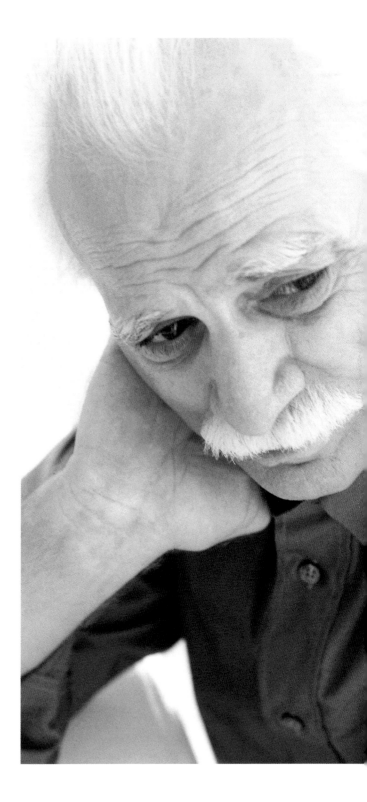

Diagnosis

There's little doubt that tinnitus is capable of driving some people to distraction. In many cases the tinnitus triggers a cycle of growing discomfort: Annoyance leads to increased attention to the noise, which builds greater frustration. Some people find the distraction so severe that they're unable to carry on with regular activities.

Several options are available that may allow you to manage tinnitus and still function in life with a reasonable degree of comfort. First, talk about the condition with your physician or audiologist. He or she can help identify or rule out a treatable cause of your tinnitus. Other specialists may become involved in the diagnosis.

If an underlying condition, such as a tumor or circulatory disorder, is causing the tinnitus, treatment may resolve the problem. Measures such as treating an ear infection or removing impacted wax also may help reduce tinnitus.

If the cause of your tinnitus remains unknown, you and your medical team can decide how best to treat your symptoms. A medical history, physical examination, hearing tests and laboratory tests may provide vital clues.

For a more detailed description of your tinnitus, the doctor may ask:
- Is one ear affected, or both? If only one, which one?
- Do you have hearing loss?
- What does the noise sound like? Is it high pitched or low pitched? How loud is it?
- Are the sounds constant, or do they change in loudness or pitch?
- What circumstances make the tinnitus better or worse?
- How does this condition affect your work habits and your ability to sleep and to concentrate?
- How has this condition affected your stress level?

An audiologist may try to determine the frequency (pitch) and intensity (loudness) of your tinnitus through audiological tests. This information can help you and your medical team select the best treatment for your situation.

Management

Though many questions remain unanswered about tinnitus, effective treatment strategies focus on managing its signs and symptoms. This focus allows you to continue functioning in your daily responsibilities and to lead a more fulfilled life.

Management may include devices such as a hearing aid or masker — or a combination of both — in addition to counseling and cognitive therapy. You and your medical team may try several approaches before deciding which one works best for you. It's often helpful to use multiple strategies.

Hearing aids and maskers

One treatment approach involves adding subtle background noise to your hearing to cover over, or mask, the sounds of tinnitus. One way to do this is by wearing a hearing aid. The hearing aid amplifies environmental sounds to make the tinnitus less noticeable. If you don't have hearing loss, or if the tinnitus is at a different frequency from your hearing loss, the device may not be as helpful in reducing the stress and annoyance of tinnitus. Hearing aids are discussed in Chapter 7.

Another way to help obscure tinnitus is a simple masker device that's worn behind or in your ear. The device resembles a hearing aid, but instead of amplifying environmental sounds, it produces low-level background noise

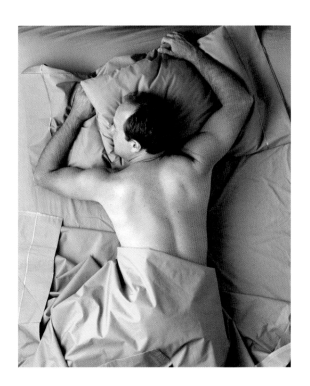

that's typically easier to tolerate than tinnitus. You have controls to adjust the loudness of the masker. Its frequency is usually programmed by the manufacturer and by your audiologist to achieve the best effect.

A third option is using a device that's a combination hearing aid and masker. This device amplifies environmental sounds but also generates background noise to help disguise tinnitus.

Often, tinnitus is most noticeable at night, when the outside world typically is quiet. Some people find it helpful to use a bedside masker (loudspeaker) to play soothing sounds, such as ocean waves, falling rain and white noise, as they prepare to sleep. This type of masker helps them relax and obscures tinnitus during periods of sleep.

To the relief of some people with tinnitus, masking can sometimes produce what's called residual inhibition. This is a period of time when your perception of tinnitus is partially or completely reduced after turning off the masker. These episodes may last from less than 30 seconds to several hours.

In certain situations, for example someone with tinnitus who also has total or nearly total hearing loss, the use of a cochlear implant may decrease tinnitus. A cochlear implant is a hearing device that picks up external sounds, bypassing the inner ear when it sends auditory signals to the brain. However, cochlear implants have also been known to cause tinnitus. See Chapter 8 for more information.

Drug therapy

If tinnitus makes you anxious or depressed, you may want to consult a physician about antidepressant or anti-anxiety medications. Although these drugs may not affect tinnitus, they may improve your outlook and help you cope with the condition.

Researchers conducted a study on the effects of the antidepressant nortriptyline on people with tinnitus — about 60 percent had experienced major depression. Results indicated that the drug helped participants sleep better and function at a higher level. The drug's side effects were rarely serious, although older adults may experience more side effects.

Studies with anti-anxiety medications also suggest that tinnitus seemed less bothersome while taking the drugs.

Most of these drugs belong to the family of benzodiazepines, including alprazolam (Xanax), clonazepam (Klonopin) and flurazepam (Dalmane). The problem is that benzodiazepines can be addictive with long-term use and are generally recommended for a period of no more than four months. Following use of this type of drug, it may be helpful to try nonmedical strategies to alleviate tinnitus.

Cognitive behavioral therapy

Cognitive behavioral therapy tries to change your understanding and perception of tinnitus rather than change the physical effects that tinnitus may have on you. This approach is based on the idea that negative thought patterns lead to negative and adverse behaviors — not unlike the cycle of discomfort and frustration mentioned before.

For example, you may be convinced that tinnitus is a sure sign of a fatal disease when, in fact, your doctor has ruled out any such possibility. A counselor trained in cognitive behavioral therapy can help you identify and examine these disturbing notions and retrain you to substitute more positive, practical thoughts.

Self-help tips for tinnitus

You may consider using these measures to reduce the severity of tinnitus and better cope with its symptoms:

Protect your hearing. Avoid loud noises, which may decrease your hearing and worsen tinnitus. If you work in a noisy environment, wear hearing protective devices regularly.

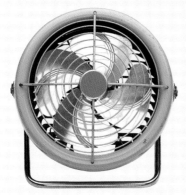

Cover up the noise. If you're in a quiet setting where tinnitus may seem more obvious, use a masker, fan, soft music, low-volume radio or commercially available sound generator to produce soft background noise that masks the tinnitus. An FM radio set between stations generates white noise. Don't use sounds that are too loud, as they may make your tinnitus seem worse and cause additional damage to your ear.

Distract yourself. Many people say they don't hear tinnitus if they're not paying attention to it. Do things that you enjoy and that absorb your attention. This will help take your mind off the tinnitus and provide needed relief.

Manage your stress. Stress can make tinnitus seem worse. The basic principles of a healthy lifestyle go a long way toward reducing stress — get plenty of sleep and exercise, and eat a healthy diet. For example, reducing tobacco, alcohol, caffeine and salt intake may help you better cope with the aggravation of your tinnitus.

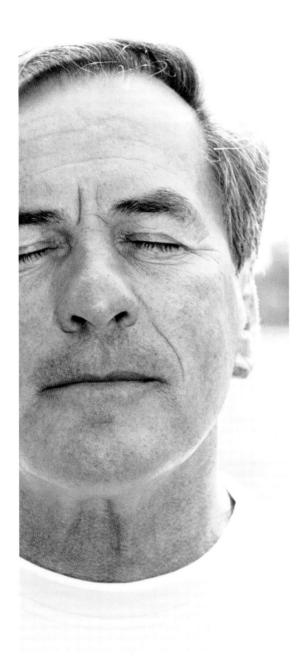

Several studies have documented the usefulness of cognitive behavioral therapy for people with tinnitus. On many occasions this approach is used in combination with other treatments, such as drug therapy or hearing aids.

Biofeedback

Biofeedback is a relaxation technique used to reduce the stress and anxiety so often associated with tinnitus. Like cognitive behavioral therapy, it aims to modify your response to tinnitus rather than alter the condition itself. You can receive training at physical therapy centers, medical centers and hospitals.

Essentially, biofeedback teaches you how to use your mind to control your bodily responses to stress. With the assistance of a variety of monitoring devices, a therapist helps you learn to control certain involuntary body responses, such as blood pressure, muscle tension and heart rate.

During a biofeedback session, a therapist applies electrical sensors to your body. The sensors monitor your response to stress — for example, muscle contraction — and feed the information back to you via sound and visual cues. With this feedback, you start associating your response — for example, headache pain — with the physical sensation of muscles tensing.

The next step is to learn how to make positive physical changes, such as relaxing those muscles, when your body is under stress. You may also be able to learn how to slow heart rate or raise skin temperature — also signs of relaxation. Your goal is to produce these responses on your own, outside the therapist's office and without the help of technology.

Biofeedback isn't for everyone who has tinnitus. Although it doesn't always reduce the perceived intensity of tinnitus, it may help you relax to the point where the noise is less bothersome. If you experience no improvement after a certain number of sessions, a different approach may be necessary.

Tinnitus retraining therapy

Tinnitus retraining therapy (TRT) is based on the idea that a person can gradually lose the awareness of a sound if that sound poses no threat or demands little attention. People can become oblivious to the sound of a ticking clock or whirring fan, even a passing train. But if the sound carries some sort of meaning with it — for example, you associate a ticking clock with being late or behind schedule — it's likely to be a sound you're most conscious of.

This concept is applied to coping with tinnitus. If you have the condition, you may have a constant urge to examine the sounds and find a cause for what you're hearing. Being unable to identify a source may leave you feeling frustrated and insecure, which further focuses your attention on the tinnitus. When this happens, it may seem as though you'll never lose your awareness of the sounds.

The goal of TRT is to get you accustomed to the tinnitus so that the persistent noise becomes just like other nonthreatening sounds and blends into the background. If the effort is successful, you'll perceive tinnitus less often on a conscious level.

To start treatment you use noise generators, usually worn in both ears, for approximately eight hours a day. The devices are set to levels that are audible but don't mask your tinnitus. You want the generators to blend the tinnitus with environmental sounds.

You'll also receive counseling that helps you perceive the condition in a rational, intelligent way so that it no longer causes fear or obsession. The audiologist will explain what's known about tinnitus and how you can become habituated to the sound.

This therapy takes time. Most people participate in the program for one to two years before stopping the use of the noise generators. Although it's not for everyone, about 80 percent of people who participated in a TRT program at the University of Maryland reported a decrease in the annoyance of tinnitus and in the amount of time they were aware of it.

Complementary and alternative treatments

Although Western science has yet to document all of the benefits and risks of many forms of alternative medicine, some people with tinnitus have reported relief with the use of vitamin or mineral therapy, herbal medicines and various dietary controls.

Other treatments that deal with the overall well-being of your body may be helpful, such as acupuncture, acupressure, yoga, hypnosis, and joint and muscle manipulation. These usually aim to reduce the general stress of life and may help reduce anxiety.

Check with your doctor before beginning any complementary or alternative treatment. Together you can determine whether it would interact negatively with any medicines you're currently taking or affect other conditions you may have.

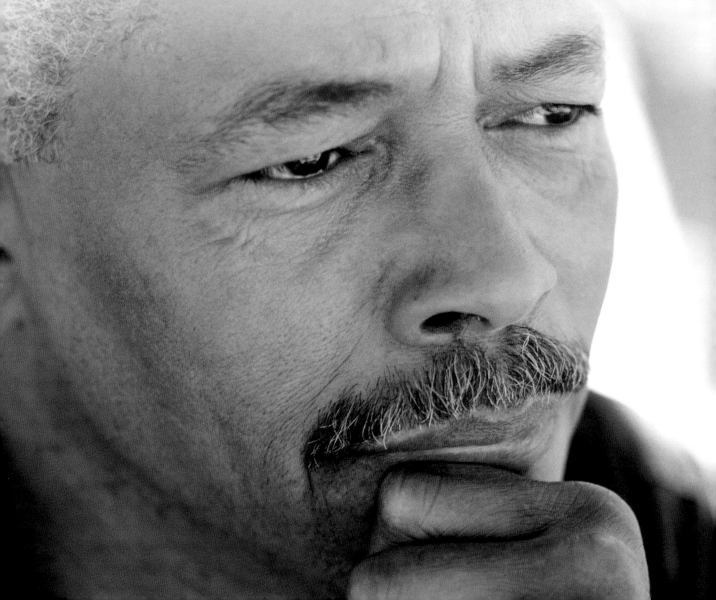

The management of hearing loss

Chapter 6

Living with hearing impairment

Hearing loss isn't a condition that you can simply ignore. It's difficult to go about the responsibilities of your daily life pretending it's not there. Hearing loss can impact your quality of life, affecting family relationships, job performance and social interactions. It can diminish self-confidence and sense of identity. For many people hearing loss is an ongoing challenge, one that may result in feeling isolated from family and friends.

But hearing loss doesn't necessarily mean your life takes a turn for the worse. You can change that trend, starting with your attitude. Acknowledging

that you have a hearing impairment — instead of denying it — is vital to overcoming its consequences.

Dealing with the challenges of hearing loss may also require changing your behaviors. Many people are uncomfortable with change and find it difficult to adjust to new routines. But learning to live with hearing loss enables you to stay engaged with family and friends and to participate in and enjoy a wide range of activities.

This chapter presents strategies you may follow to improve your ability to communicate and find emotional and financial support. Assertive communication, speech reading and sign language also may help you. In addition, the chapter directs you to support groups and community resources.

Quality of life

Sound helps anchor you to the outside world. Sound gives you pleasure and a sense of belonging. Sound also alerts you to danger or opportunity.

Hearing impairment may deprive you of listening to the laughter and conversation between friends at a social gathering or the inspiring sounds of nature on a forest trail. Activities such as eating at a restaurant, traveling, attending religious services, classes or concerts, and watching movies become more difficult. Even something as routine as talking on the telephone, shopping for groceries and running errands can pose special challenges.

Frequently, hearing loss is gradual over several years. For that reason it may take time to recognize that you're having more difficulty hearing. In fact, family and friends may notice your hearing loss before you do.

Initially you may deny or try to minimize the hearing impairment, perhaps because you can still hear certain sounds well. You may convince yourself that other people only need to speak more clearly or slowly. But denying your hearing difficulties or blaming them on external factors doesn't make the problem go away.

Access

Have you ever strained to understand what's being said over a public address system? Have you found yourself unable to enjoy the theater because you can't hear the actors unless they speak in your direction? Have you struggled with schoolwork because the classroom either mutes or echoes the teacher's voice? Situations like these can be stressful for anyone in an active life. They present unique challenges for people with hearing impairment.

All too often, people with hearing impairment aren't provided with the communication tools they need for travel, entertainment, education and medical care. Few movie theaters provide captioning services or assistive listening systems. Many medical clinics and hospitals don't have interpreters on staff for the hearing impaired.

In denial

Why do so many people deny having hearing loss? And why do so many put off getting help — sometimes for years? Denial happens for many reasons:

- Hearing loss develops gradually, so you may not recognize the problem at first. Often, you find ways to compensate for hearing loss without even being aware that you're doing so. For example, you may become very adept at speech reading without realizing it.
- Many people underestimate the severity of their hearing loss. When people lose their hearing, they tend to lose their ability to hear high-pitched tones first, such as the consonant sounds. Consonants are the sounds of speech that provide clarity and crispness to what you hear. Voices may still sound loud, but they also seem unclear.
- People often associate hearing loss with old age. You may fear the stigma of wearing hearing aids.
- You may fear being considered incompetent. A common concern expressed by people coming to terms with hearing loss is that others will assume they're also losing their ability to think and act independently.

When you're in denial about hearing loss, you're not able to admit to yourself that there's a problem. You may convince yourself that you heard what was said or that you just weren't paying attention. You may deflect attention from your hearing loss with expressions such as "You're mumbling again" or "I don't need to hear what they're saying" or "I'm too young for hearing aids."

Whatever the cause, denial won't help you for the long term. If you can't admit to hearing loss, you'll have trouble taking the steps to communicate better and make life easier. You'll only prolong the time it takes for making adjustments and finding solutions.

Organizations such as the Hearing Loss Association of America (HLAA) are working to improve access in a variety of situations for people who are hearing-impaired. Improvements in assistive technology are allowing more hearing-impaired people to participate in a greater range of activities. The advent of online learning has improved access to education. For more information about assistive listening devices, captioning and other communication aids, see Chapter 9.

Employment

Hearing impairment may cause problems at work. You may misunderstand a conversation with your manager because of background noise in the office or shop. You may have difficulty hearing someone speaking to you through a glass partition, such as at a teller's window, or from another room. You may have trouble participating in meetings or conferences with several people talking rapidly at once.

Practical solutions to many common workplace problems such as these are available. It's also useful to know your legal rights. Almost every state has a statute making it illegal to discriminate in employment on the basis of disability, race, religion, sex, age or other minority status.

Under the Americans With Disabilities Act (ADA), it's against the law to discriminate against qualified people with physical and mental disabilities in job application procedures, hiring, firing, advancement, compensation and training. You can find more information about these important regulations at the Department of Justice Web site (www.ada.gov).

The ADA requires employers to make what's called reasonable accommodation for employees with disabilities. A reasonable accommodation can be any modification or adjustment to a work environment that enables the employee with a disability such as hearing loss to perform essential functions of the job.

For deaf or severely hearing-impaired employees, reasonable accommodations may include providing a telecommunications device for the deaf (TDD), captioned telephone, videophone or even something as simple as a flashing ringer on the regular telephone.

Sound barriers or muffling can be added to office walls and floors to control background noise in the work

Dealing with hearing loss in the workplace

You'll benefit from the adjustments your employer can make to create a more accessible environment, but you too can take steps to reduce potential problems in the workplace:

- Use the communication aids that are provided. These may include assistive listening devices such as telephone amplifiers, FM systems, captioning and alerting devices. These resources are discussed in Chapter 9.
- Move away from the source of background noise. If possible, locate your desk away from busy hallways and noisy office machines, such as air conditioners and photocopiers.
- Ask co-workers to address you by name as they speak. This allows you to focus your attention, understand what's being said and participate in discussions.
- Sit upfront at meetings and presentations. Arrive early or ask to be seated close to the speaker.
- Give yourself a break in between situations that require a lot of listening and communication. Try not to schedule meetings one after the other. Otherwise fatigue may set in.
- Alert co-workers to situations that may cause problems. Let them know how they can help you communicate.

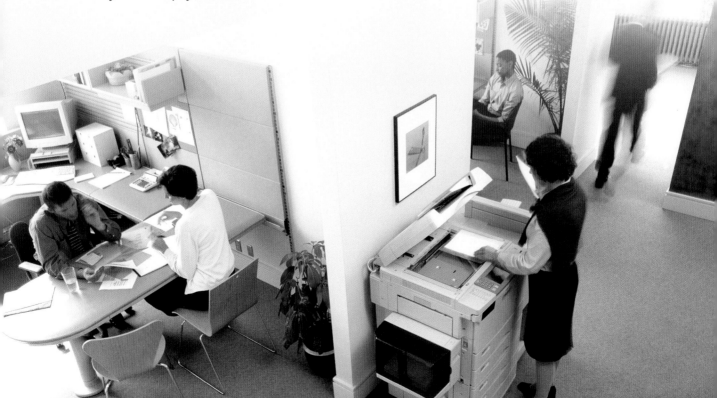

environment. Assistive listening systems can be installed in auditoriums and meeting rooms. The services of a transcriber or sign language interpreter can be sought out. In addition, employers should change or add lighting to enhance visibility.

State governments operate vocational rehabilitation agencies to help people with disabilities retain their present jobs or, if that's not possible, retrain for other jobs. Rehabilitation means getting ready for useful employment and successful integration into society. Certified rehabilitation counselors and rehabilitation psychologists can help address your work-related concerns.

Relationships

Humans are social creatures — most people seek out connections with others and thrive on them. Living in an intensely social world can be difficult when your ability to communicate is hampered. Hearing loss can strain your relationships with family, friends, co-workers and anyone with whom you interact regularly.

For example, when you're unable to hear much of what's being said at a dinner party, you may tire quickly from the effort and feel left out. This may cause you to skip these events and stay home. At the store you may have trouble hearing your charge total from a soft-spoken clerk. If your spouse calls to you while you're working in front of a running faucet or dishwasher, you may not understand the words.

Factors associated with hearing loss, such as social isolation, low self-esteem and depression, may further strain these relationships.

Isolation. When you're struggling to hear, conversations quickly become frustrating and tiresome. Although you want to spend time with your family and friends, interacting gets too stressful. It's natural to try to avoid situations that you know will be difficult. In so doing, you may cut yourself off from the world around you and the people who love you.

Social isolation is a serious problem for older adults with hearing impairment. Research by the National Council on Aging found that hearing-impaired older adults who don't use hearing aids are more likely to withdraw socially, become depressed, and feel that other people get upset and angry at them for no reason.

By contrast, hearing-impaired older adults who use hearing aids tend to have a higher quality of life, better relationships with their families and better feelings about themselves. They're more socially active, experience more interpersonal warmth, and have greater emotional stability.

To minimize the negative effects of hearing loss, it's important to remain socially involved. Casual conversations with friends, attendance at family gatherings, dinner parties and card games, and evenings at the movies or theater — these are pleasurable activities that keep us involved in the mainstream of life. Strategies to improve communication and social interaction are discussed starting on page 124.

Identity. Hearing loss affects how you perceive your place in the world. Many adults whose hearing loss occurred early in life have, over time, incorporated the impairment into their self-image — they perceive themselves only in this way. As a result they're more accustomed to managing hearing loss in their daily lives and routinely cope with it.

For adults who experience hearing loss late in life, the impairment can be more

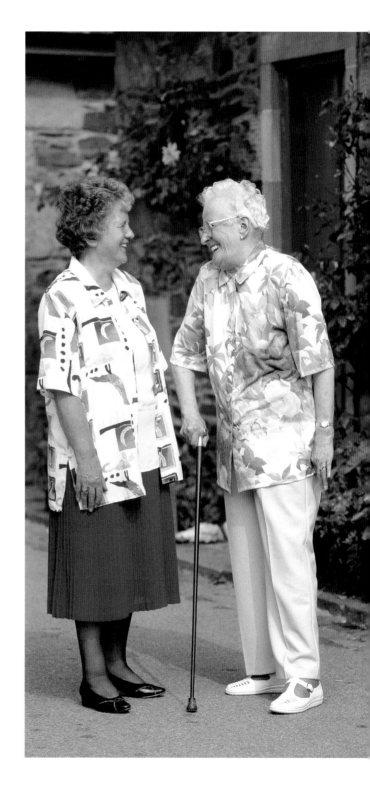

disturbing and disruptive. Commonly, feelings of inadequacy accompany hearing loss and inhibit daily activities. Hearing loss may be considered a social stigma. They fear that others will treat them as incompetent.

To build your new identity as an adult with hearing loss, you may need to let go of some preconceived notions about aging and focus on the positive aspects of your life.

Emotional effects

Everyone's experience with hearing loss will be slightly different. But most people who endure any kind of serious loss — whether it's physical or emotional — go through the stages of denial, anger, bargaining, depression and acceptance. Other feelings associated with loss include frustration, embarrassment and sadness.

Two common emotional effects of hearing loss are depression and anxiety.

Depression. Depression isn't a weakness, nor is it something that you simply "snap out of." Depression is a medical condition that affects how you think and behave and can cause many emotional and physical problems.

Individuals who are depressed often deny or minimize the problem — which only delays treatment and can make the problem worse. Signs and symptoms don't always follow a particular pattern. But they can include persistent sadness and feelings of hopelessness, loss of appetite, sleep disturbance, extreme mood changes, irritability and poor concentration.

Many studies have demonstrated a link between hearing loss and depression. Compared with peers who have normal hearing, older adults with hearing loss report significantly more signs and symptoms of depression. Most individuals experiencing the condition will improve following treatment involving both medication and counseling.

It should be noted that depression is often considered a natural stage in the grieving process. In other words it may represent a part of coming to terms with your hearing loss. Regardless, you should not delay seeking medical treatment for the condition.

Anxiety. Anxiety involves extreme worry and fear about a future event, whether or not it's likely to happen. The feeling often stems from misinformation and mistrust of the unknown.

Anxiety can be influenced by other factors, including family history, personality and general outlook on life. Anxiety and depression often go hand in hand.

Signs and symptoms of generalized anxiety include restlessness, irritability, impatience, muscle tension, sleep problems, headache, shortness of breath and difficulties with concentration.

Hearing loss sets the stage for many anxiety-producing situations: On the way to a store, you may be anxious about understanding the cashier. When going to meet a friend, you may fear that you'll misunderstand the conversation. On your own, you may be concerned about hearing warning sounds of danger, such as traffic noise or the footsteps of someone approaching around a blind corner.

Research shows that as hearing loss progresses from a mild to moderate level, anxiety increases as well. People with hearing loss may develop deep anxieties toward social situations in which they believe it will be difficult to hear clearly. They tend to avoid these situations at all costs.

If you're concerned that you or someone you care about may have an anxi-

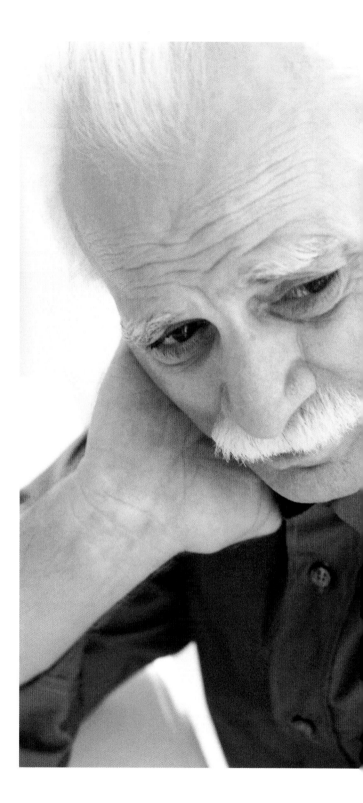

ety disorder, talk to your doctor or a mental health professional. Treatment can help you manage the condition.

Improving social interaction

Although hearing loss may change your relationships with others, many strategies and tools can allow you to still communicate effectively and stay involved in a range of activities.

As you're learning new communication skills, you may work with health care professionals, other people with hearing loss, family and friends. Most people are eager to help you communicate better. But you must be more than a passive recipient of their services — learning requires your commitment and effort.

Effective communication can occur even if you don't hear each and every sound. Your remaining hearing, along with visual information, context clues and life experience, help you understand speech. With the assistance of technology, the impact of hearing loss can be considerably reduced.

Assertive communication

Good communication may require you to become more assertive. But being assertive doesn't mean being loud and intrusive. Assertiveness simply means letting others know your needs without ignoring their needs in the process. Often, without some assertiveness, you may not be able to hear and understand anything in a conversation.

Assertive communication means being forthright about what it will take for you to participate and interact. With assertive communication, you:

- Let others know that you have hearing loss. Then they won't misconstrue your behavior or think you're aloof or forgetful.
- Are aware that your hearing loss affects other people and are prepared to deal with their reactions.
- Are willing to use hearing aids and assistive listening devices.
- Ask for, but not demand, help when you need it.
- Tell people exactly what you need. You might ask individuals to slow their speech, look at you when they speak or move a hand from their face, or repeat a phrase.
- Take a break from conversation when you're tired.

- Show your appreciation when others make an effort to communicate better with you.
- Are willing to admit if you're taking out your emotions on others.
- Modify your environment to fit your hearing needs.

With assertive communication, you'll probably find it easier to cope with many social situations. Most people will be receptive if you tell them you're having trouble hearing and will ask what they can do to help.

Creating an environment for better listening

One of the most effective strategies for better hearing and social interaction is to modify situations that make listening difficult. Often, by altering or stage-managing your environment, you can avoid communication breakdowns. Following are suggestions that might help you:

Move closer to the source of a sound you want to hear. This may include a television or stereo system, a public speaker or lecturer, or a visitor to your home. Arrange furniture so that guests or family members are nearby and facing directly toward you. In locations

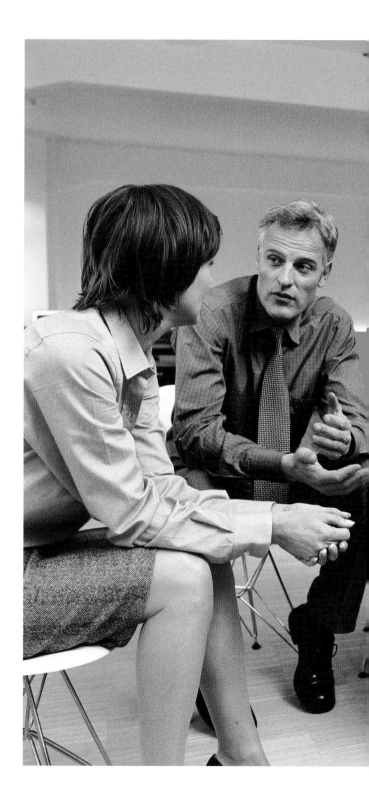

Communicating with a hearing-impaired person

Communication is the lifeblood of any relationship. When you're conversing with someone who's hearing-impaired, keep in mind that what to you is simple communication may be a tiring effort for your companion. He or she has to make an active effort to understand. Hearing aids may help, but turning up the volume won't make distorted sounds any clearer.

You can enhance communication with a hearing-impaired person by following a few practical suggestions:

- Before starting to talk, reduce the level of background noise. Turn off the television, radio, air conditioner or other noisy appliances. Don't leave a faucet running. If you can't reduce background noise, try to move to a quieter area.
- Make sure you have the person's attention before speaking. You can do this by saying his or her name or touching his or her shoulder.
- Talk face to face. Speak at eye level, and no more than a few feet away. Don't chew gum, smoke, talk behind a newspaper or cover your mouth while you're having the conversation.
- Speak at a normal conversational level, especially if the person is wearing hearing aids or has a cochlear implant. Don't shout. If necessary, modestly increase your volume.
- Speak clearly but naturally. Slow your speech a little, using a few more pauses than usual.
- Use facial expressions, gestures and other body language to make your points.
- Watch your listener's face for signs that comprehension is a problem. Rephrase your statements if the listener is unsure of what's been said.
- Alert your listener to changes in topics of conversation.
- Show extra consideration in a group situation. What's known as cross talk is one of the most difficult situations for someone with hearing loss. Try to structure the event so that only one person is speaking at a time. At meetings it's helpful to display an agenda on a board or overhead transparency and, as the meeting progresses, to indicate which item is under discussion.

where you can't rearrange furniture, choose your seating for minimum distance and maximum visibility.

Move away from distracting or overpowering noise. When you're in public places, try to avoid sitting in locations close to machinery, appliances or busy hallways. In a restaurant, request a table away from the kitchen, lobby, bar or other noisy spot, and sit with your back to the wall. Avoid sitting close to music speakers or ventilation ducts.

At home, turn off or mute the television or radio when you're conversing with someone. Seat yourself away from open windows that let in traffic noise and outdoor sounds.

Position yourself so that the speaker's face is visible and well lit. Visual cues, such as facial expressions or the position of the head, provide clear indications of what's being said. Good lighting helps your speech reading.

Plan in advance for social activities. Before attending an event in a busy or crowded setting, such as a theater or place of worship, call ahead to see if the facility is equipped with assistive listening devices. Arrive early so that you have a choice of seats.

Speech reading

Speech reading, also called lip reading, is a tool that individuals with hearing loss can use to navigate many social situations. With this technique, you learn to recognize spoken words by watching the movements of the speaker's lips, tongue, lower jaw, eyes and eyebrows, as well as facial expressions, body stances and gestures. These visual cues are critical for understanding.

Most people, whether they hear normally or not, rely on speech reading to some degree. In fact, many individuals are unaware that they can speech read. For example, when background noise is extremely loud, people with normal hearing may try instinctively to match the motion of the speaker's lips to the sounds they hear.

Speech reading works best if you still have some hearing ability left and use hearing aids or other assistive devices. It's accomplished primarily by following lip patterns — the shapes made by people's mouths when they speak. For example, the vowel *o* is formed with rounded lips, the consonant *m* is made by pressing the lips firmly together, and the consonant *l* requires placing the tongue behind your teeth.

But even the most skilled speech reader can't pick up every word. Not all sounds are visible on the lips, and some sounds look exactly alike. For example, the consonants *b, m* and *p* look similar on the lips. So the words *ban, man* and *pan* are almost impossible to distinguish.

Other factors — rapid speech, poor pronunciation, bad lighting, averted face, covered mouth, facial hair — can make speech reading more difficult. You often need to rely on the context of the sentence and other nonverbal cues to understand what's being said.

As with any new skill, learning the basic techniques for speech reading takes time and patience. For people with hearing loss, including those with hearing aids, speech sounds may be muted or distorted. And you must learn to focus on the lip movements.

But your skill usually improves with practice, and the more you practice, the more confident you'll become. Many proficient speech readers find that the technique allows them to follow conversations more easily. Some people who are profoundly deaf choose to communicate using speech reading and speech rather than sign language.

Tips for speech reading. Rather than trying to catch every word that's spoken, focus on the overall intent and context. Here are other suggestions for making speech reading easier:

- Position yourself so that a light source is behind you and the speaker's face is clearly visible. Any factor that reduces the visibility of the lips will interfere with your ability to speech read.
- Identify the topic being discussed as quickly as possible. If you're familiar with the topic and can identify key words, you won't need to analyze every phrase.
- Watch for clues in the speaker's facial expressions, body language and gestures.
- Before you enter a conversation, inform the person who's speaking that you have hearing loss. Ask the person not to shout, exaggerate mouth movements, chew gum or talk rapidly.
- Try to relax as much as possible. Don't try to understand everything, or you may become tense, which can only make speech reading that much more difficult.
- Use your remaining hearing in combination with speech reading. Diminish background noise by turning off the television or radio,

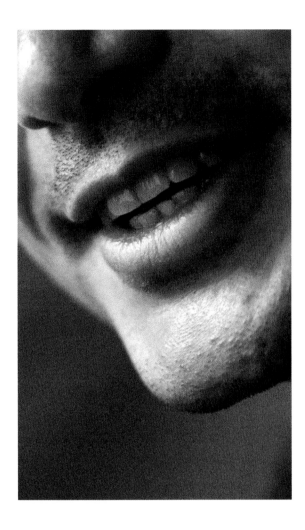

• Take frequent breaks, especially when you're first learning to speech read. The technique requires deep concentration, and you may tire quickly from the effort. When you get the chance, close your eyes and relax for a few minutes.

Cued speech

Another useful technique that can help people with hearing loss to listen and communicate is known as cued speech. This system supplements the basic principles of speech reading (lip movements) with the use of "cues" — specific hand shapes and hand placements around the mouth.

The eight hand shapes represent different consonant sounds. The placement of the hands represents vowel sounds. So, by combining a hand shape and hand placement, you create a visual cue for an individual syllable. Using this technique in combination with lip reading can greatly improve your understanding and communication.

Cued speech was developed as a way to improve literacy in children with severe hearing impairment. Its success is due to making the sounds of spoken language look different.

closing the door or window, or sitting in a quieter section of a restaurant, away from the bustle.
• Focus on the message rather than specific lip movements. You'll find that subsequent sentences may clarify the words you've missed.
• If you can't fill in a missing word, ask the speaker to rephrase the sentence in a different way.

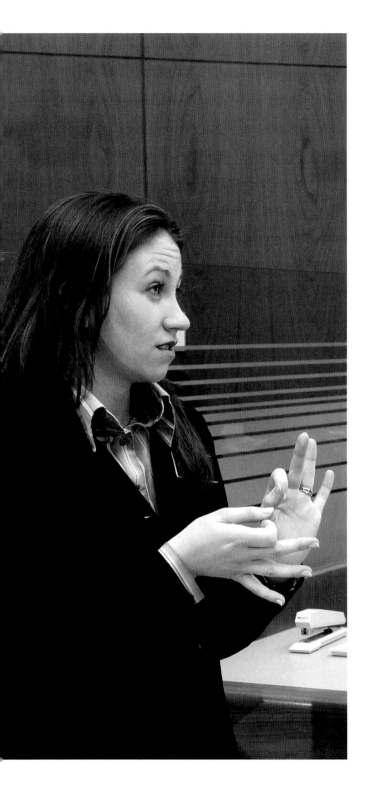

Sign language

Sign language uses hand signs — made with hand shape, position and movement — as well as body movements, gestures, facial expressions and other visual cues to form words. It's often the first language of many individuals who are deaf or have severe hearing impairment.

Sign language is a complete language with distinct grammar, semantics and syntax. This is unlike cued speech, which is based on the sounds and structure of a spoken language.

Different sign languages are used in different countries and regions of the world. American Sign Language (ASL) is commonly used in the United States and Canada — in fact, it is the fourth most commonly used language in the United States. And like the English language, ASL allows for regional differences and jargon.

Sight is considered the most valuable tool for using sign language. Each sign in this language may be broken down into parts — in the same way that spoken words can be broken down into individual sounds and intonations. Each ASL sign is, in fact, a distinct combination of hand shape, hand movement and hand location. Changing any one of these parts changes the meaning of the sign.

Facial expressions and body movements also are very important in sign language. For example, English speakers usually signal that they are asking a question with a raised tone of voice. ASL users ask a question by raising their eyebrows and widening their eyes. Stating a command may require them to sign more emphatically.

Learning sign language. Using sign language takes time and practice, and learning from a book is difficult. It's generally recommended that you enroll in classes and meet with other people who use sign language. Picking up enough signs for basic communication can take a year or more of training.

Community colleges, universities, libraries, continuing education programs and vocational rehabilitation centers are some of the institutions that may offer sign language classes. The American Sign Language Teachers Association (ASLTA) certifies qualified teachers. The ASLTA Web site (www.aslta.org) has information about state and local chapters.

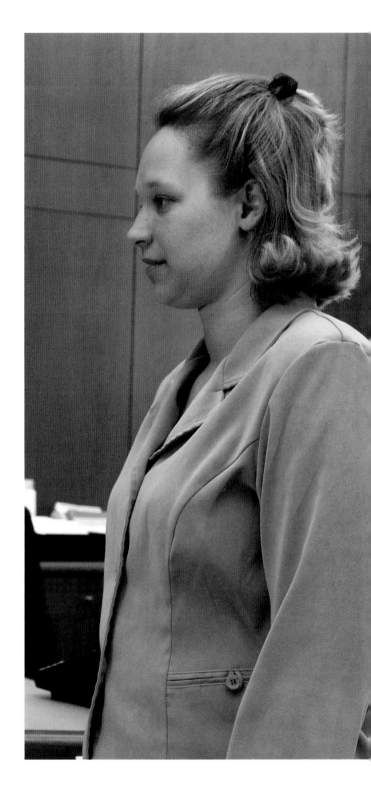

Hearing dogs

You're probably familiar with guide dogs for people who are blind. Did you know that service dogs are also available to help people with severe or profound hearing loss? Hearing dogs can alert you to everyday sounds such as a doorbell, ringing telephone, oven timer, alarm clock and smoke and fire alarm. A dog can even respond when someone calls your name.

Hearing dogs don't bark to get your attention. Rather, they're trained to use their nose or paw to nudge you, then lead you to the source of the sound. Hearing dogs can also carry messages or notes between you and another household member.

Paying attention to your hearing dog's reactions in public spaces can help you be more aware of car traffic and pedestrians, especially when they approach you from behind or around a corner.

According to the Americans With Disabilities Act, hearing dogs must be allowed to accompany their owners into businesses and other places that serve the public. Often a bright orange or yellow leash identifies a hearing dog. But the dog doesn't have to have special identification to accompany you into a business or public space.

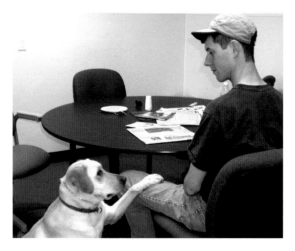 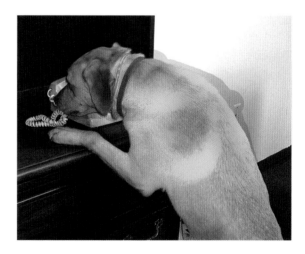

Helpful hearing dog

To alert you to a sound, a hearing dog will first nudge you to get your attention (left), then lead you to the source of the sound, such as a ringing telephone (right).

Getting a hearing dog. Hearing dogs come in all shapes and sizes. Many are taken from animal shelters and given three to six months of training — obedience training as well as special service training. There's no national training standard, and the dogs aren't required to be certified.

Some people with hearing loss choose to participate in the training, working directly with a private trainer and the dog. Others prefer to get a dog that's already trained. Regardless, you may have to wait two or more years before getting a canine companion.

In the United States, the two largest hearing dog organizations are Paws With A Cause and Canine Companions for Independence (CCI). Most service-dog organizations are nonprofits that provide the dogs at no charge to the people who need them.

Finding support

Even under the best circumstances, living with a hearing impairment will have frustrating moments. There will be times when you feel overwhelmed by the effort of staying connected to the hearing world or isolated by your inability to hear certain sounds.

You don't have to cope with all of the challenges alone. Various options are available that provide support to people with hearing loss, such as aural rehabilitation or a support group. Many national, state and local organizations provide information on preventing hearing loss and resources for living with hearing impairment.

Aural rehabilitation

If you don't feel comfortable with your hearing impairment, consider aural rehabilitation, also called hearing rehabilitation or auditory training. Aural rehabilitation helps you adjust to hearing loss and tries to reduce the difficulties. Advocates say that by making the best use of hearing aids and assistive listening devices, you can take charge of your communication needs.

An audiologist, a speech-language pathologist or both typically provide rehabilitation services. You may work one-on-one with a therapist or as part of a group or in both settings. Group therapy can be especially helpful because you'll meet others facing the same issues as you are.

Evaluating information

You can find hundreds of products, publications, services and Web sites devoted to hearing impairment. But be careful. The information ranges from solid research to outright quackery.

When evaluating information you find on the Internet, consider these guidelines:

- Look for Web sites created by national organizations, universities, government agencies or major medical centers.
- Search for the most recent information you can find.
- Check for the information source. Notice whether articles refer to published research. Look for a board of qualified professionals who review the content before it's published. Be wary of commercial sites or personal testimonials that push a single point of view.
- Double-check the information. Visit several sites and compare the information offered.

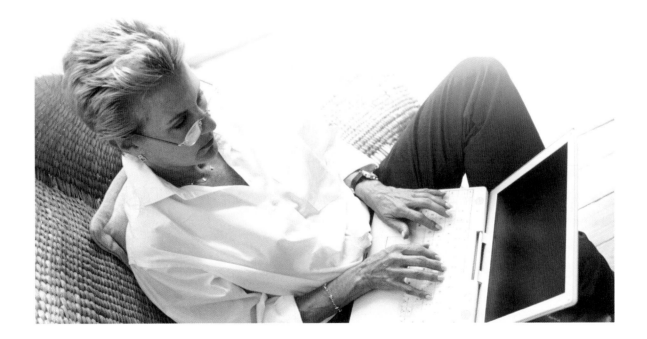

The overall goal of aural rehabilitation is to maximize self-confidence and your ability to communicate with others in everyday situations. This can be achieved by:

- Understanding your hearing loss
- Learning how to listen
- Learning skills in speech reading
- Building confidence in communication situations
- Dealing with emotional problems related to hearing loss
- Learning about all the options among different hearing aids and assistive listening devices
- Understanding your legal rights and being your own advocate
- Promoting your family's understanding of your needs
- Making it easier for your family to communicate with you

A typical rehabilitation session lasts from one to two hours a week. The session may be held at a medical clinic, rehabilitation center, community college or private office. Aural rehabilitation sessions generally last over a period of four to 10 weeks.

There are now commercially available aural rehabilitative software programs that can be used at home and at your own pace of learning.

Support groups

Sharing experiences with other people with hearing impairments is a great way to find support. Belonging to a group can remind you that you're not alone in dealing with this problem.

Support groups aren't the same as group aural rehabilitation. An audiologist leads an aural rehabilitation group. Peers frequently lead support groups.

Support groups are an excellent resource for problem solving and mutual support. They're also a way to meet potential new friends. How have others handled traveling, meetings, telephone conversations, communicating in public places or dealing with difficult work colleagues? What problems have they had with hearing aids? Have they used assistive listening systems?

Many national organizations with local chapters provide support groups for people with hearing loss. These include the Alexander Graham Bell Association for the Deaf and Hard of Hearing, the Association of Late-Deafened Adults, the Cochlear Implant Association, the National Association of the Deaf, League for the Hard of Hearing, and Hearing Loss Association of America

(HLAA). See "Additional resources" at the back of this book for contact information for these organizations.

National, state and local resources

Dozens of national, state and local organizations provide services for people who are deaf or hard of hearing. These resources include advocacy, education, financial aid, referral, advice on medical issues, and counseling on professional and work issues.

There are also opportunities for self-help and support groups, recreational and social activities, and spiritual needs. Most organizations have Web sites and publications about hearing loss that offer easy-to-understand information for the public.

The federal government provides information on affirmative action programs, reasonable accommodation and improving accessibility for disabled persons. For example, if you feel your legal rights have been violated, you may contact the Equal Employment Opportunity Commission for advice.

States provide services for individuals who are deaf and hard of hearing. The state office might be a commission or vocational rehabilitation program for people with disabilities. Offices that provide rehabilitation services often provide counseling and job retraining and may help pay for hearing aids.

Some states have programs to provide amplified telephones to people with hearing impairment. A state human rights or human relations commission or a governor's committee on employment of people with disabilities can provide information on related laws.

Chapter 7

Hearing aids

Hearing loss doesn't mean you're cut off from the world of sound. But you may need a little help to make the sounds you hear audible and understandable. If you feel like you're missing out because of hearing loss, you'll likely benefit from a hearing aid.

Hearing aids are sophisticated electronic devices that make sounds louder. They don't restore your hearing to what it was, but they can improve your ability to listen and communicate in daily activities. Hearing aids are the single most effective treatment for a majority of people with hearing loss.

Hearing aids can greatly enhance personal interactions. They minimize many problems associated with hear-

ing loss, such as difficulty understanding conversations — face-to-face or on the telephone — and being aware of signals, timers and beepers. Hearing aids can help combat feelings of social isolation and problems with self-image.

Hearing aid technology has improved tremendously in recent decades. Many years ago hearing aids were large and cumbersome. They had a harsh, distorted sound quality, like that of a cheap transistor radio. Newer hearing aids are compact and provide far better sound quality. Many options are available to match your lifestyle and your communication needs.

As you adjust to a new hearing aid, you'll start to enjoy your improved ability to hear and communicate in a variety of social situations. You may feel a little safer when you can hear environmental sounds around you. You'll likely notice improvements in your quality of life by regularly wearing the aid and taking good care of it.

Setting priorities

Motivation is the key to success with hearing aids. People with a positive attitude and commitment to hearing better are often the best hearing aid users. They're also more likely to continue wearing the devices.

There are a variety of hearing aid styles. Selecting which type to use is often a personal choice based on your specific needs — each person and each type of hearing loss is quite different. In making the selection, it helps to be informed, patient and open to the suggestions of your audiologist and hearing aid dispenser.

There are several things you can do to increase your satisfaction with hearing aids. You've probably already taken the first steps — acknowledging your hearing loss, having your hearing tested, and seeking out the best solutions to the challenges this loss presents.

It's also important to know what you can realistically expect from a hearing aid. Identify the situations in your life when communication is most difficult. When are the times when it's important for you to hear especially well? Are there occasions when you have to concentrate so hard on hearing that you become fatigued? Perhaps you want to make sure you can hear your children or grandchildren when they visit, or to understand conversations during a weekly card game.

When considering which type of hearing aid to buy, you'll typically face trade-offs among many factors, such as performance, style, size, technology and cost. For example, you may simply want the smallest device available. Or maybe you prefer a hearing aid that's easy to operate, regardless of size.

If you're retired and spend most of your time at home, the most expensive brand with all the latest technology may not be required. Prepare a list of priorities, ranking the various considerations by their order of importance.

Resistance to hearing aids

Despite the benefits of hearing aids, many people with hearing loss haven't ever bothered to try one. Studies indicate that only about 24 percent of the estimated 31 million Americans with hearing loss use a hearing aid. People reject the notion of wearing an aid for many reasons, including an unwillingness to accept hearing loss, cost of the device and reports of bad experiences with hearing aids from friends or relatives. Often the biggest deterrent is fear of the social stigma — concern that a hearing aid is a sign of old age, incompetence or unattractiveness.

Such concerns have little basis in fact. Studies have examined whether hearing aids actually do make people look older. The conclusions were that, indeed, hearing aids might make the wearers look older — but by less than one year, a difference so small as to have no practical significance.

In addition, the advances in technology and design are making hearing aids stylistically more appealing and functionally more effective. Each improvement, big or small, seems to have only increased user satisfaction with the devices.

Weigh the benefits of hearing aids against the obstacles of being unable to understand what people are saying. You'll need to accept that a hearing aid isn't a sign of aging and dependence. The device will enhance your communication with others, increase your independence and help you stay socially connected and involved.

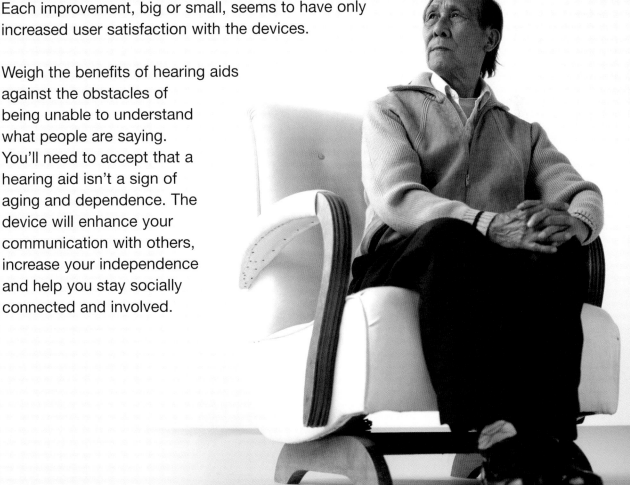

Everyone experiences varying degrees of success with hearing aids. How well they function for you personally will depend on many variables, including the type and severity of your hearing loss. But if you expect a hearing aid to restore perfect hearing, you're bound to be disappointed.

One way to develop realistic expectations is by educating yourself about your type of hearing loss. Another is by talking to other people who have coped with hearing loss. It's also important to work closely with an audiologist or hearing aid dispenser.

How hearing aids work

There are many types of hearing aids available, and the technology is continually improving. But the fundamental purpose of all hearing aids is the same: to make sounds stronger and thus more audible. They allow more sounds to be heard.

Hearing aids collect sounds from the environment via a small microphone. They amplify these sounds and then direct an amplified signal into the user's ear via a speaker. The amplified signal stimulates the inner ear, activating nerve fibers that carry the sound impulses to your brain.

The illustration on the adjoining page labels the parts of what's known as an in-the-ear style of hearing aid.

With hearing aids, you should be able to understand words spoken in conversation without needing to strain as much. They should make it easier for you to hear people talking in a soft voice. You'll probably be able to turn down the volume of your television to a level that's more comfortable for others in the room who don't have hearing loss. Hearing aids can also help you hear environmental sounds, which gives you a better sense of what's taking place around you.

Hearing aids may help you in situations where you previously had difficulty hearing, such as a theater performance or worship service when the speaker is far away or the sound is weak. They can help you feel more at ease when you're on your own — for example, while shopping — or in situations where speakers may not be talking directly to you.

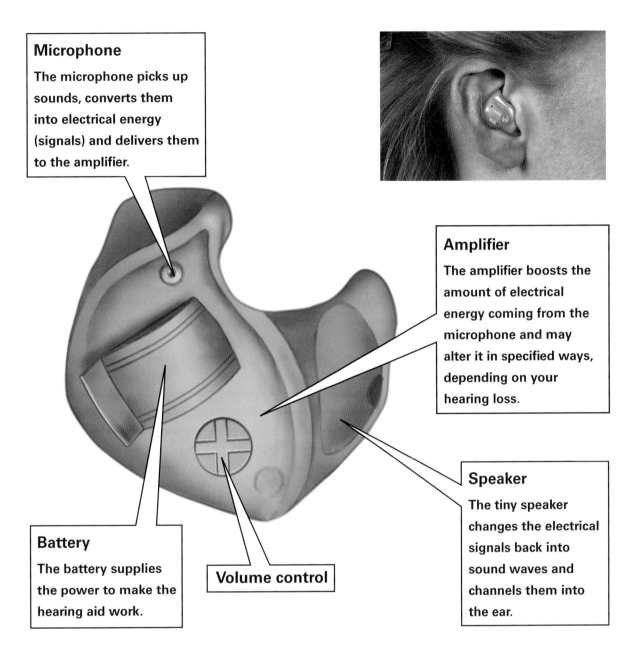

Microphone

The microphone picks up sounds, converts them into electrical energy (signals) and delivers them to the amplifier.

Amplifier

The amplifier boosts the amount of electrical energy coming from the microphone and may alter it in specified ways, depending on your hearing loss.

Speaker

The tiny speaker changes the electrical signals back into sound waves and channels them into the ear.

Battery

The battery supplies the power to make the hearing aid work.

Volume control

Parts of a hearing aid

All the components of this in-the-ear style of hearing aid are held in a small plastic container called the casing. In a behind-the-ear style of hearing aid (see page 145), the casing rests behind the ear and is connected to an earmold by a plastic tube. The earmold is custom fit to direct sound into your ear canal.

Hearing aids may improve your hearing, but they don't provide a completely natural sound. They're electronic devices, after all, which can slightly change the quality of what you hear — just as a radio might slightly change the quality of music being played.

When you first listen through a hearing aid, you may notice that many things sound a little different. But you'll likely adapt to this change quickly.

Furthermore, hearing loss typically causes the ear to distort some of the sounds you hear. Hearing aids can't eliminate that distortion, so those sounds may not be crystal clear.

You may continue to have problems understanding speech in certain situations. For example, when there's background noise or many people talking at once, hearing aids can't isolate the voice that you want to hear from other sounds. Remember that even with normal hearing, background noise frequently interferes with your understanding of speech.

Some newer hearing aids have added features that may help you in difficult listening situations. These attachments are discussed on pages 149-150.

Selection

When selecting a hearing aid, your decisions primarily involve different styles, sizes and circuitry features. You may also be faced with choosing whether one or two devices are necessary to improve your hearing. This process can become confusing because the decisions regarding style, size and circuitry can be made somewhat independently of each another.

For example, you may have heard that digital hearing aids provide the best sound. What may not be clear is that *digital* refers to the electrical components and not to a particular style of hearing aid. Style and circuitry — along with size — are separate issues. Any circuitry can be placed in any style or size of hearing aid.

Hearing aid electronics

The circuitry of hearing aids refers to the electronic components inside the casing. Hearing aid electronics are specially programmed to amplify certain frequencies more than others. And the frequencies that are programmed correspond to the locations in your cochlea where hair cells are damaged.

Are two hearing aids better than one?

Can you hear better with a hearing aid in each ear? The answer, in most cases, is yes. Wearing two (binaural) hearing aids has many advantages over wearing one (monaural) aid. More auditory information is sent to your brain, and the signals reaching each ear will be slightly different. This makes it easier to hear speech in situations where there's background noise.

Two aids also provide more balanced hearing. You won't have a bad side, where sound is muted. Having two ears to listen with helps you locate the origin of sounds more easily, so you won't have to turn your head around to figure out who's talking. Another advantage of wearing two aids is that neither device needs to be turned up as loudly as when you're wearing only one. This helps reduce feedback and increases comfort.

Financial constraints and inability to wear an aid in one ear keep some people from wearing two aids. Talk to your audiologist about your options.

Nearly all of today's hearing aids contain a small computer chip — so they're referred to as digital hearing aids. This type of aid converts incoming sound into a digital code, which is analyzed and adjusted based on your hearing loss and listening needs. Then the code is converted back into sound waves and delivered to your ear canal.

Computer chips provide many new options in sound processing and make the devices more comfortable for use in various sound environments.

The computer chip allows the audiologist to program your hearing aid to fit both the objective characteristics of your condition as well as some of your own subjective preferences. For example, the chip allows the audiologist to adjust how much amplification is required for you to hear at different ranges of frequency and pitch. This will depend on the type and severity of your hearing loss.

In addition, the computer chip can allow for several different settings for amplification. The audiologist can program one setting for use in quiet situations and another setting for use in loud, noisy situations such as restaurants or parties. You can select which setting you want by pushing a small button on the outside edge of the hearing aid or, in some cases, with the use of a remote control.

Often, special features in the circuitry can be activated for use in certain settings. For example, in noisy situations, you can activate directional microphones in the hearing aid that reduces the amount of noise that's picked up behind you — typically, background noise. Special noise reduction circuitry may also be included.

With some aids, the computer chip itself can automatically adjust the settings based on the amount of noise and on how loud the sounds are.

Some hearing aid circuitry allows devices worn in the right ear and the left ear to communicate with each other to make joint setting adjustments. Furthermore, hearing aids are being developed that incorporate wireless technology, permitting better communication between the hearing aids and cell phones or other electronic devices.

Digital hearing aids are available across a wide price range, from relatively inexpensive to very expensive. The cost is determined primarily by how many special features and adjustments are included on the computer chip. For many users, the less expensive aids may contain enough features to suit their hearing loss and their lifestyle. Other users may prefer to include all possible features and are willing to pay for them accordingly.

Hearing aid styles

Hearing aids come in various styles, which differ in size and the way in which they fit in the ear. Some aids are small enough to fit deeply in the ear canal, making them almost invisible. The most widely sold aids are those that fit behind the ear — accounting for approximately half of all the hearing aids that are dispensed.

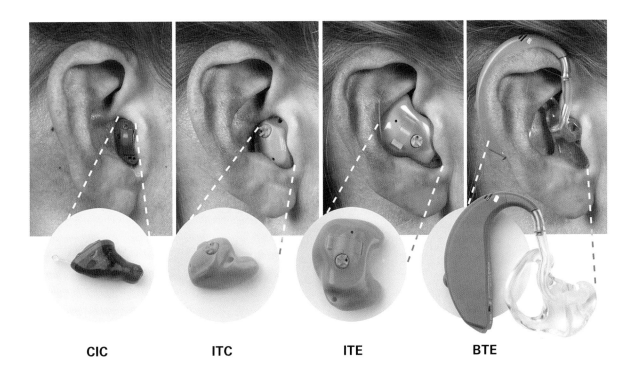

Hearing aid styles

Styles include completely in the canal (CIC), in the canal (ITC), in the ear (ITE) and behind the ear (BTE). All styles can be equipped with digital circuitry, although the smallest, least visible CIC style cannot be equipped with many add-on features.

In general, the smaller a hearing aid is, the less powerful it is, the shorter its battery life and the more it will cost. Smaller aids are more likely to produce feedback. Feedback refers to a high-pitched whistle and crackle that occurs when amplified sound is inadvertently picked up by the microphone and re-amplified. This is similar to the noise you may hear over a public-address system when the volume is too high. New technology is helping to reduce feedback problems in hearing aids.

With different styles to choose from, keep in mind that the choice of a hearing aid concerns more than just looks. The style that may best suit you will depend largely on your hearing test results. Usually, the greater your hearing loss, the larger your hearing aid will need to be.

Also, some styles of hearing aids tend to not work as well when your hearing remains good at the low frequencies but decreases substantially at the higher frequencies.

The size and shape of your outer ear, especially the ear canal, may eliminate certain style options. For example, in-the-canal styles can be difficult to fit in smaller ears. In addition, your ability to handle a small hearing aid may be a factor if you have limited finger dexterity. Medical conditions also may dictate which style is appropriate.

Completely in the canal. The smallest hearing aid available is called a completely-in-the-canal (CIC) aid. All parts, including the battery, are contained in the tiny casing that fits deep inside the ear canal. A thin, plastic pull cord on the aid sticks out into the bowl-shaped part of your ear to help in removal. The CIC aid is appropriate for mild to moderate hearing loss. It's not used for children or infants.

Advantages. This is the least visible hearing aid. It may help reduce problems with wind noise.

Disadvantages. This is the least powerful style and not suited for severe hearing loss. CIC aids have less space for options such as volume control or directional microphones. In addition, the batteries are small, so battery life will be shorter. It's susceptible to problems with earwax clogging the speaker and microphone openings.

In the canal. An in-the-canal (ITC) hearing aid fits partly in the ear canal but not as deeply as a CIC aid. The outer edge of the ITC aid extends into the bowl of your ear. ITC aids can accommodate mild to moderately severe hearing loss, but they're not appropriate for use with infants and children.

Advantages. Like CIC aids, ITC aids are hardly visible. An ITC aid is likely to be more powerful than a CIC aid, with more opportunity for add-ons.

Disadvantages. Like CIC aids, ITC aids can be difficult to handle and insert into the ear, and for replacing batteries.

In the ear. An in-the-ear (ITE) hearing aid fills most of the bowl-shaped area of your outer ear. It's also known as the full-shell style. ITE aids are suitable for mild to severe hearing loss.

Advantages. ITE aids are more powerful than smaller aids, and they can accommodate more options, such as a telecoil and directional microphones (for more on options, see pages 149-150).

They're appropriate for a wider range of hearing loss. The battery may be larger and easier to insert than batteries for the in-the-canal styles.

Disadvantages. ITE aids may pick up more wind noise than may the smaller in-the-canal styles.

Behind the ear. Behind-the-ear (BTE) aids have two parts. A small plastic casing that rests behind the ear contains the hearing aid circuitry: the microphone, amplifier and speaker.

The casing is connected by plastic tubing to a custom-made earmold (earpiece) that directs the amplified sound into your ear canal. BTE aids are suitable for almost all types of hearing loss and for people of all ages.

BTE aids are often perceived — erroneously — as old-fashioned and not technologically advanced. In fact, BTE aids contain the latest digital technology like the other styles and may offer the greatest improvement in hearing.

Advantages. These are the most powerful hearing aids available, and they can be programmed for any level of hearing loss. There's also plenty of space for options. BTE aids are the best style for infants, children and people with severe hearing loss. BTE aids are also the easiest devices to maintain, partly because battery replacement is easier. These aids usually require fewer repairs than other styles.

Disadvantages. Some individuals simply don't have enough space between their ear and the side of their head to accommodate a BTE aid. This style may pick up more wind noise than the smaller aids do.

Open fit behind the ear. A recent style that has become popular for mild hearing loss is the open-fit-behind-the-ear hearing aid. This is a smaller version of the behind-the-ear style. Typically, the casing is completely obscured behind the outer ear. A very thin tube connects the casing to the ear canal, leaving the canal still largely open — hence the name "open fit."

An open-fit aid works well for individuals with relatively good hearing at low frequencies and mild to moderate hearing loss at higher frequencies.

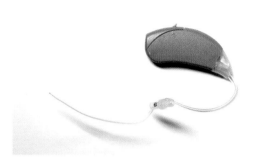

Open fit behind the ear

This hearing aid style is well suited for individuals with mild to moderate hearing loss. Because the ear canal remains open, users can continue using their remaining hearing for lower pitched sounds.

However, people with more severe hearing loss can't use the open-fit style because of inadequate volume.

Because most of the ear canal is open, individuals can use their remaining hearing for lower pitched sounds — which are able to pass directly to the eardrum — and the hearing aid selectively amplifies the higher pitched sounds.

Advantages. The ability of the small casing to fit inconspicuously behind your ear, and the use of very thin tubing, makes the open-fit style very attractive to individuals who have cosmetic concerns. Leaving the ear canal open often makes the individual's own voice sound more acceptable.

Disadvantages. Due to the open ear canal, this style is limited in how much volume it can produce before feedback problems occur.

Bone anchored. The bone-anchored hearing aid (BAHA) is attached directly to your skull and stimulates the inner ear via bone conduction. The BAHA system is best used for mild to moderate conductive hearing loss. It can also be used in certain cases of severe to profound unilateral hearing loss (in one ear but not the other).

A titanium post is surgically implanted into your skull. A microphone and amplifier, both within the same external casing, are attached to the post.

Advantages. BAHA aids can be used when more conventional hearing aids that use air conduction cannot function. For example, when there's a physical abnormality or chronic drainage from the ear that makes the use of earmolds a problem. A BAHA aid is more comfortable than other types of bone-conduction hearing aids.

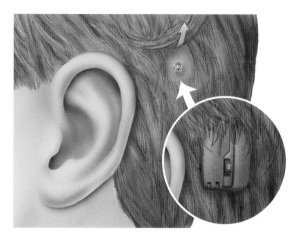

Bone anchored

An external microphone and amplifier attached to a titanium post surgically implanted in the skull transmits sound via bone conduction.

Disadvantages. Surgery is required to implant the titanium post. Any repairs to the device may be costly.

Implantable. Implantable hearing aids may be an option for people with moderate to severe sensorineural hearing loss, that is, loss associated with damage to the inner ear.

These devices use a tiny electromagnet attached to the bones of the middle ear and an external unit that stimulates the magnet. This type of aid is rarely used and has not worked particularly well.

Special options

Other considerations when choosing a hearing aid are options that can help you in difficult listening situations.

Directional microphones. Most hearing aids are equipped with an omnidirectional microphone, which picks up sounds from the side and behind as well as in front of you. That's generally a good thing until you're trying to hear someone in situations where there's a lot of background noise, such as in restaurants or places of employment.

A directional microphone picks up the sounds directly in front of you more than the sounds coming from other directions. This can diminish the background noise processed by your hearing aid, and improve your understanding of face-to-face conversations.

A hearing aid may have a microphone with dual sound inlets or be equipped with multiple microphones. Either arrangement allows you to switch between directional and omnidirectional modes. In fact, many hearing aids are equipped to make this switch automatically as the acoustic environment changes. All but the CIC aid can have directional microphones.

Telecoils. Many BTE hearing aids, as well as some ITE and ITC aids, contain a built-in telecoil circuit. A telecoil is a tiny metal rod encircled with a coil of copper wire. The coil generates an electric current when it receives naturally produced electromagnetic signals from the telephone receiver. The hearing aid converts the current into sound, allowing you to hear clearly when someone talks to you on the telephone.

The telecoil can be manually activated with a switch, but many hearing aids now have an internal switch that picks up the electromagnetic signal automatically. When the telecoil is switched on, the microphone in your hearing aid is turned off and only the telecoil signal is amplified. This avoids the feedback or squeal that often happens when a telephone is held close to a hearing aid with the microphone switched on.

Besides telephones, telecoils can be used with assistive listening systems (see Chapter 9). Telecoils may not work with cell phones that are not hearing-aid compatible.

Remote control. Some hearing aids can be operated with a remote control device. This feature allows the user to turn the hearing aid on or off, and to adjust settings without touching the hearing aid or trying to find a small button or knob on the casing.

Audio input. An input jack on the aid allows you to connect a wire directly to a television, stereo, separate microphone or assistive listening device.

Ear-level FM systems. FM listening systems are particularly helpful for overcoming the impact of background noise, reverberation and distance on your hearing (see Chapter 9). Some BTE hearing aids combine regular circuitry with an FM receiver in the same casing. The receiver responds to a direct signal from the FM transmitter.

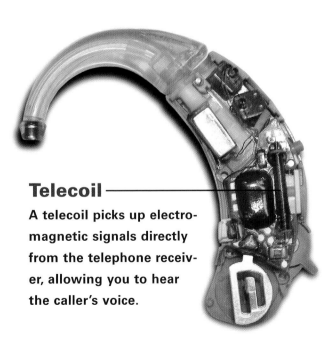

Telecoil

A telecoil picks up electromagnetic signals directly from the telephone receiver, allowing you to hear the caller's voice.

Buying a hearing aid

If you're planning to use hearing aids, you'll want to consult first with an audiologist or a hearing aid dispenser, also known as a hearing instrument specialist.

Audiologists have a graduate degree in audiology, are certified by either the American Speech-Language-Hearing Association or the American Academy of Audiology, and are licensed by the state in which they practice. The practices of many otolaryngologists include audiologists on staff to provide testing and rehabilitation services and to dispense hearing aids.

Although hearing aid dispensers aren't required to have a college degree in order to practice, many have completed coursework in the field. They're registered in the state they work in. Most states require hearing aid dispensers to be licensed, which means that they've passed state-administered written and practical examinations in the field. Dispensers should be certified by the National Board for Certification in Hearing Instrument Sciences.

It's important to find a reputable and qualified hearing aid dispenser. Start by asking your doctor for recommendations. In addition, you can get lists of hearing aid dispensers in your area by contacting professional organizations such as the American Academy of Audiology, the American Speech-Language-Hearing Association and the International Society of Hearing Instrument Specialists.

Several Internet sites that sell hearing aids will refer you to dispensers within their network — but this practice is illegal in several states. Don't buy hearing aids by mail or over the Internet from makers who claim you don't need to see a dispenser in person.

Discuss hearing aid options thoroughly with your audiologist or hearing aid dispenser. Make sure you understand why a specific type of hearing aid has been recommended and how it can meet your needs.

Regardless of which type of hearing aid you buy, always purchase it with a return privilege. The aid should come with a 30- to 60-day trial period and a return policy. You may use that time to adjust to using the device and decide whether it helps your hearing.

Purchasing tips for hearing aids

Keep the following suggestions in mind when selecting a hearing aid:

- Considering all the options available, more than one type of hearing aid might work for you. If your first selection is unsatisfactory, try a different type.
- Don't assume that the newest, most expensive model is also the best — a less expensive aid might improve your hearing just as much.
- Be cautious of "free" consultations and dispensers who sell only one brand of hearing aid. Look for a dispenser who offers plenty of options.
- Be alert to misleading claims. Be wary of advertisements that claim hearing aids can eliminate background noise or restore normal hearing. Most aids can help you, but no hearing aid can completely filter out one voice from other voices or restore your hearing to normal.
- Ask what the cost of a hearing aid includes. Most dispensers offer a single fee that bundles the cost of the aid with the costs of follow-up visits, the warranty and one pack of batteries.
- Get the terms of the trial period and the warranty in writing. This should include the return policy, the amount that can be refunded, how long the warranty lasts (preferably one or two years) and specifically what is or isn't covered — the warranty should cover both parts and labor.
- During the trial period, keep a detailed list of what you like or dislike about your hearing aid. Take the list with you when you return to the dispenser.

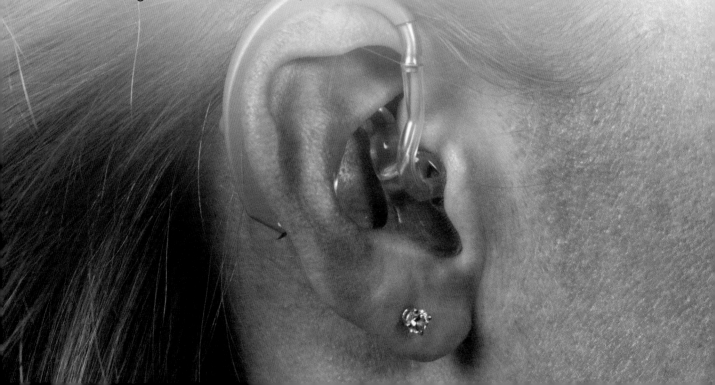

The buying process

In the discussion that follows, the terms *hearing aid* and *aid* are used in the singular form. But keep in mind that frequently the most improvement results from a hearing aid in each ear.

To start the process, plan on being examined by a physician, preferably an ear, nose and throat specialist. The Food and Drug Administration (FDA) requires hearing aid dispensers to obtain proof that you've had a hearing examination within the past six months before they can sell you a hearing aid, or you'll have to sign a waiver.

The hearing examination helps decide whether any medical treatment can improve your hearing or if a condition prevents you from using a hearing aid. Although few health insurance plans pay for hearing aids, many that offer coverage require a medical clearance prior to purchasing the device.

Also schedule a complete hearing evaluation by an audiologist. Get a copy of your audiogram if you're not buying a hearing aid at the same place where you've been tested. The audiogram provides an accurate guide for selecting the hearing aid.

Discuss all of your needs and expectations with the hearing aid dispenser. Indicate which situations cause you the greatest amount of difficulty with hearing. Your goal is to match your lifestyle and your communication needs as closely as possible.

After studying the evaluation of your hearing loss and your lifestyle needs, the dispenser will discuss various options with you and offer some recommendations. Before you make a final decision, make sure you're aware of all the features included, as well as the cost of your selection and the terms of the trial period and return policy.

After you've made a selection, the dispenser will need to fit the hearing aid. For most types of aids, the dispenser makes an impression of your ear, using a putty-like material to create an accurate mold of its shape. This mold helps the manufacturer make a hearing aid that's comfortable and fits properly in your ear.

After one or two weeks, you'll return to the dispenser's office to resume the fitting with your actual hearing aid. This visit also involves programming the aid to provide maximum assistance for your hearing loss.

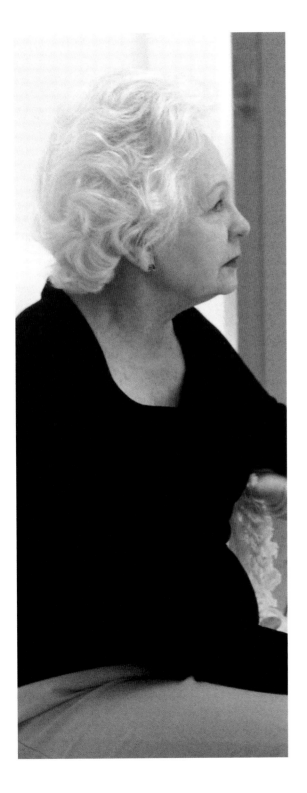

Once the aid is fitted, the dispenser should instruct you on how to operate and maintain the hearing aid — how to insert and remove the device, check the battery, adjust the controls and keep it clean and operational.

The trial period allows you to adjust to the hearing aid. You'll probably schedule a return visit to the dispenser within a few weeks. Until that time, write down questions or concerns and take them with you to the appointment.

If during the trial period you can't adjust to the aid or you decide that your hearing doesn't benefit enough from its use, notify your dispenser. Under the agreement, you're entitled to a refund for the cost of the device.

Costs

The cost of a hearing aid varies considerably. Most digital aids range from $800 to $3,000. Your costs will be about double if you get two aids. Although this may seem expensive, if hearing aids can help you hear better and improve your quality of life, they're worth the investment.

Medicare and most private insurance policies don't cover the cost of a hearing aid. A few employer- or union-sponsored policies provide limited reimbursement. Qualified veterans may be eligible for free hearing aids and services through the Veterans Affairs. Some fraternal and charitable organizations provide financial assistance for hearing aids for people who meet financial eligibility requirements.

Wearing your hearing aid

You should notice immediate improvement in the first days of wearing a hearing aid, but more benefits for your hearing come after you've become more accustomed to using the device.

Getting used to a hearing aid takes patience and practice. Your brain requires time to readjust to sounds that you may not have heard for a while. Some sounds will seem different when they're amplified by the device.

To get the maximum benefit from your hearing aid, it's important to understand how it works, learn to insert it properly and use it regularly. A positive attitude also helps.

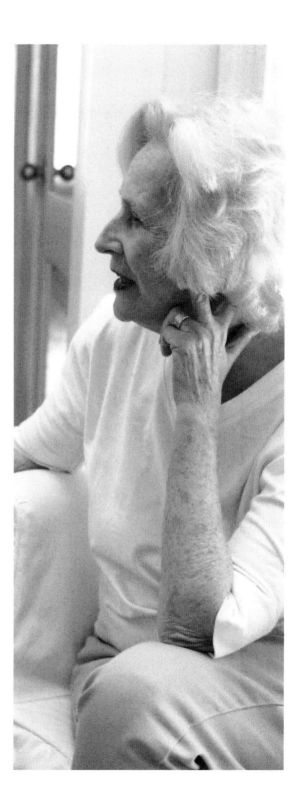

Schedule return appointments. After you've had your hearing aid for a week or two, you may wish to have it adjusted for more or less loudness or for better fit and control. The audiologist or hearing aid dispenser will help you achieve the best possible fit and greatest benefit for your hearing.

The audiologist or hearing aid dispenser will continue to counsel you on operating and maintaining the aid. Practice using the device in his or her presence. If you use two aids, insert and remove both to learn how to distinguish between the device for your right ear and the one for your left ear. Practice adjusting the controls, cleaning the aid and changing the batteries.

Readjustment

When you first use a hearing aid, some sounds may not seem natural. You may have come to think of what you hear with hearing loss as normal. Now, with the use of an aid, you're exposed to more sounds and louder sounds, as well as different patterns of sound.

Many first-time users of hearing aids say that other people's voices, as well as their own voices, sound strange. In fact, the voices you hear are being

picked up by a microphone and amplified. Hearing aids are often programmed to amplify certain pitches more than others depending on your type of hearing loss — so you may be hearing pitches that you haven't heard for some time. However, the more you wear the aid, the quicker the sounds will seem normal to you.

As your hearing has decreased over the years, you've probably become more accustomed to a quieter life. Many common environmental sounds, such as appliance motors, clocks, dripping faucets, a car's running motor, footsteps, even your own chewing or breathing, were soft or inaudible when you weren't using a hearing aid.

During the first months of wearing a hearing aid, you'll start noticing these sounds again. Because you haven't heard them for a while, your brain is more aware of them. The change may annoy you. But after several months, your brain will shift these sounds to the background where they belong, and you'll notice them less.

Many hearing specialists recommend that new hearing aid users build up their listening experiences gradually, wearing their aids for only a short time in quiet situations. New users often make the mistake of immediately wearing hearing aids in the most difficult listening conditions, such as loud restaurants. Starting off in this way can be frustrating and discouraging.

If you're having a problem adjusting to the aid, consider using it only for a few hours a day in your home, where you can control the noise level. Practice conversing with one or two people in a quiet place. Gradually increase the amount of time you use your hearing aid each day.

As your comfort level builds, expose yourself to different listening situations

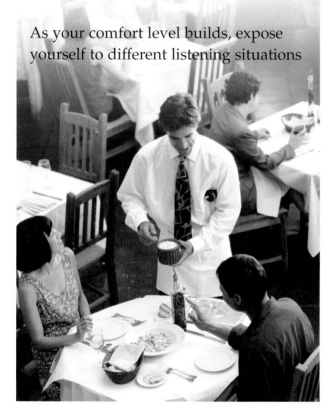

until you're able to use your aid all day in any environment. It will take some time, perhaps months, to get used to new sounds and achieve the maximum benefit from your hearing aid.

Discuss any problems you experience with your audiologist or hearing aid dispenser. You may be directed to a group orientation session for new hearing aid users. This session provides information about hearing loss and hearing aid use. You may also contact an organization such as the Hearing Loss Association of America.

Remember that hearing aids are meant to improve communication, not to give you new ears or the normal hearing of a healthy 20-year-old. You'll inevitably encounter circumstances in which hearing aids don't give you all of the benefits you'd like. In these situations you may rely on other methods for improving communication.

Tips for better communication

Difficult listening situations may require you to use other, simple techniques in addition to your hearing aid. Consider these strategies to improve your hearing in these circumstances:

Hearing aid batteries

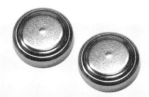

Use only the size and type of battery recommended by your hearing aid dispenser. Most hearing aid batteries are zinc-air. They're activated when an adhesive tab is removed and air gets into the battery. Never remove the tab until you're ready to insert the battery into your hearing aid. Zinc-air batteries have an excellent shelf life, so you can keep several packages on hand. Store them at room temperature, not in a refrigerator.

Battery life depends on the style and circuitry of the hearing aid, the size of battery and how many hours a day the aid is used. Most hearing aid batteries last from one to two weeks, although small batteries last only about three to seven days. Discuss a battery replacement schedule at your initial fitting.

You can buy batteries from your audiologist or hearing aid dispenser, or in drugstores, grocery stores and electronics supply stores. Make sure to keep them out of reach of children and pets, and dispose of them properly.

Talk face to face. Supplement what you hear with what you see. When you're talking to someone, make sure you can see his or her face and lips. Converse on a one-to-one basis or in small groups rather than large groups.

Don't talk to people from a different room. Distance and physical barriers such as walls reduce the amount of sound that reaches you.

Control background noise. Talk in locations with the least background noise. Steer clear of noisy restaurants, or go during off-peak times to avoid a crowd. You may also ask for a booth in a quiet corner with good lighting. In meeting rooms and lecture halls, sit in the front row. At home, turn off the television or stereo while conversing on the telephone or in person.

Ask others to help. People are usually glad to accommodate you if they understand your needs. Let others know how to help you and what listening strategies work for you. Start by telling people that the circumstances are making it difficult for you to hear. Ask them to talk directly to you face to face and to speak clearly, but it's not necessary to shout.

Educate yourself about other assistive tools, including devices and listening systems. Resources such as a telephone amplifier, FM transmitter, induction loop or closed captioning service may prove helpful in difficult listening environments. These resources are discussed in Chapter 9.

Common problems

As with any complex piece of equipment, things can go wrong with a hearing aid. Most hearing aid problems are minor and easily corrected.

It's always important to inform your audiologist or hearing aid dispenser of any problem. Before calling the dispenser, however, check to make sure the problem isn't something that you can easily fix:

- Is the hearing aid turned on?
- Are all switches or controls in the correct position?
- If you have a remote control for the aid, is it functioning?
- Is the sound outlet plugged with wax or debris?
- Is the microphone opening plugged?
- Is the battery fresh and inserted properly?

The following lists some of the most common problems with hearing aids, and ways for solving them.

Feedback. Discordant sounds such as whistling and squealing are usually the result of a poor fit, an improperly inserted device or an ear plugged with wax. The more powerful a hearing aid is, the more critical the fit. When you experience feedback, always check for the following:

- Make sure the aid is inserted properly in your ear.
- Make sure the volume control isn't set too high.
- Have your audiologist or doctor check your ear for wax buildup.

If feedback continues to be a problem, you may need to check if your hearing has changed. When in doubt, have your ears examined and hearing tested.

Dead or defective batteries. Weak and faulty batteries are a leading cause of hearing aid failure. Signs of a failing battery include weak output, distortion, increased feedback, and strange or unusual sounds, such as crackling static or fluttering.

If any of these signs become evident, try inserting a new battery. Make sure that the battery is placed correctly with the plus and minus signs facing in the right direction. Many new hearing aids will give you a warning tone that your battery soon needs replacing.

Wax blockage. Placing a hearing aid or earmold in your ear canal seems to stimulate wax production. People who don't wear hearing aids can also get wax buildup, but it gradually loosens, moves to the edge of the ear canal and falls out. The hearing aid or earmold can compress the wax and cause it to stay in the canal. The wax can block the speaker and shut it down.

The best way to prevent wax buildup is to visit a doctor or audiologist regularly to have the wax removed. It's a simple procedure. Don't try to remove the wax by yourself using cotton swabs. This may only pack the wax deeper into the ear canal and damage your eardrum.

Ask your hearing aid dispenser about a means to keep wax from getting inside your hearing aids, such as a wax guard. Every day, inspect the end of the hearing aid where the sound comes out and look for wax blockage. Ask your dispenser to show you the best way to clean wax from the aid.

Ear discomfort. The earmold of a BTE aid or the shell of smaller aids should fit snugly but not uncomfortably in the ear. Initially, the earmold or hearing aid may feel slightly uncomfortable, but it shouldn't cause soreness, redness or irritation. Discomfort may also result from a poorly fitting aid or from an aid that's positioned incorrectly in the ear canal. Difficulties with correct placement are fairly common among many new hearing aid users.

If you experience constant discomfort from wearing a hearing aid, consult your hearing aid dispenser about the problem. The earmold or hearing aid may need to be modified or remade.

Moisture. BTE hearing aids have the most problems with moisture because the casing is farther away from the ear canal. Moisture often collects in the tubing between the earmold and the casing — as warm air from the inside of your ear travels into the cooler tubing, water vapor condenses and collects in the tubing. Condensation usually isn't a problem unless the tubing becomes plugged. Storing the aids in a dehumidifier pack may help.

where someone has just taken a shower, and don't spray it with hair spray.

Check the small holes at the tip of the hearing aid. Clean out any wax with a small brush, a wire looped around the end of a piece of plastic (a wax loop) or a pick. Consider getting a built-in wax guard on your hearing aid.

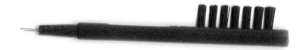

Maintenance

Proper care is a key to keeping your hearing aid in good working order and ensuring that it'll last as long as possible. Following are suggestions for maintaining your hearing aid:

Keep your hearing aid clean and dry. Wipe your hearing aid with a tissue or soft cloth every time you take it out of your ear. Gently scrub it with a soft brush every evening when you're finished using it for the day. A dry, soft-bristle toothbrush works well.

Don't wear your aid while bathing, showering or swimming. Keep it away from steamy kitchens or bathrooms

Keep the hearing aid in safe, dry, dust-free storage. You may want to buy a dehumidifying container to store it in at night. Ask your dispenser to recommend a container that would work for you.

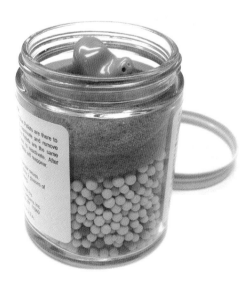

Don't expose the hearing aid to intense heat. Don't leave the aid on the top of a radiator, and don't leave it in the car in the sun.

Open the battery door when the hearing aid isn't in use. This ensures that the hearing aid is turned off. It also lets dry air in and moisture out.

Don't drop the hearing aid. Develop the habit of inserting and removing your aid over a soft surface, such as a bed or sofa. Never leave the aid where it could be knocked to the floor.

Have the hearing aid cleaned and serviced regularly. Never repair a hearing aid yourself. This can damage the aid and void the warranty. If the hearing aid breaks or malfunctions, contact your hearing aid dispenser.

Always keep the hearing aid and the batteries away from small children and pets. They can choke on an aid or swallow a battery.

Chapter 8

Cochlear implants

Sensorineural hearing loss involves damage to the inner ear and to the auditory nerve that connects with the brain. The damage is often permanent and the hearing loss irreversible.

One of the most promising treatments for adults and children with severe to profound sensorineural hearing loss is a cochlear implant. A cochlear implant is an electronic device that generates a sense of sound for people who would get little or no benefit from the amplified sound of hearing aids.

A cochlear implant is something like an artificial inner ear, taking over the job of the cochlea. A healthy cochlea converts sound waves into electrical signals and sends those signals along the auditory nerve. If the cochlea is damaged, an implant can be surgically placed in the inner ear that directly stimulates the auditory nerve. It's activated by a device worn outside the ear.

Research on cochlear implants began in the 1950s as scientists looked to help people with sensorineural hearing loss. They began experimenting with ways to compensate for the damaged hair cells in the inner ear.

Cochlear technology has evolved in sophistication and is still improving. Tens of thousands of adults and children in the United States and around the world have benefitted from the procedure and are using the implant in their daily lives.

Although a cochlear implant doesn't restore normal hearing, it can dramatically improve your ability to hear and to understand speech. Benefits from the implant vary from person to person, but some users find that it allows them to perform many routine tasks such as talking on the phone or listening to classroom lectures.

Hearing with a cochlear implant is different from normal hearing and takes time to learn. But after using a new device for a few weeks or months, the recipient usually finds that the sound of other voices begins to seem natural. For children with hearing loss since birth or a very young age, cochlear implants can help them acquire speech, language and other essential developmental skills.

Many recipients of cochlear implants feel that their quality of life improves following the procedure. The new sense of sound helps reduce feelings of isolation and increases their ability to participate in many social situations. They're able to enjoy pleasurable sounds such as the laughter of babies and the harmonies of song. They feel safer because they can hear fire alarms, warning sirens and traffic noise. They can better perform their jobs by being able to hear the ring of a telephone or the beep of a timer and to participate more at one-on-one or group meetings.

Cochlear implants and hearing aids

A cochlear implant is very different from a hearing aid. Hearing aids amplify sound waves, making them stronger when they're delivered to the ear canal. This amplification helps make more sounds detectable, louder and understandable to a damaged ear.

A cochlear implant doesn't make sounds louder. Rather, it bypasses the damaged or nonworking parts of your inner ear and directly stimulates the auditory nerve. The implant gathers acoustic information from your environment and converts it into a form that your brain can understand.

Normally, the sensory hair cells in your cochlea convert sound vibrations arriving from the middle ear into nerve impulses. These impulses are relayed to the brain, which interprets the

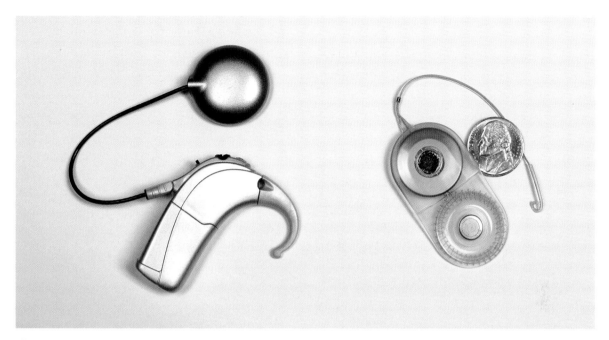

Cochlear implant

A cochlear implant includes an external component, at left, made up of a microphone, speech processor, and transmitter. The component at right is implanted into your skull and connected directly into the cochlea. The nickel is included only as a size reference.

impulses and gives them meaning as sounds. For example, the brain might receive nerve impulses for the word *yellow.* With normal hearing, your brain would understand the word as *yellow*, but with hearing loss you might misinterpret the sound as *jello.*

In order for a person to hear sounds correctly, thousands of tiny hair cells must be functioning in the inner ear in order to fully detect the vibrations. A person with normal hearing will typically have 20,000 to 30,000 healthy, delicate hair cells in each ear.

In most people with sensorineural hearing loss, some of the hair cells are damaged and don't function properly. They're unable to stimulate the auditory nerve. Although many nerve fibers are intact and able to transmit electrical impulses, these fibers are unresponsive because of the hair cell damage.

People with mild or moderate hearing loss still have a sufficient number of healthy hair cells. Sounds that are amplified by a hearing aid can be converted into electrical impulses by the undamaged hair cells, in the same way that sounds are transmitted in a normal-hearing ear.

But if you have severe to profound sensorineural hearing loss, extensive hair cell damage prevents your auditory system from processing the information, no matter how much hearing aids amplify the sound.

Cochlear implants help resolve this sensorineural problem because they're able to stimulate the intact nerve fibers directly. This allows you to still communicate auditory information to your brain and perceive sounds.

How cochlear implants work

Different cochlear implant systems are available. The Food and Drug Administration (FDA) has approved several systems and is doing clinical investigations to test others.

All systems work by converting sounds into electronic impulses that are transmitted to your brain. The implants aren't single units — they have both internal and external components. The external components are a microphone, speech processor, transmitter and connecting cords. The internal components are a receiver-stimulator and electrodes. These parts work together as follows:

- The microphone picks up sounds from the environment. It's located in a headset or casing that's hooked over the ear, similar to a behind-the-ear hearing aid.
- The speech processor is a small, powerful computer chip that digitally converts the sounds from the microphone into electronic impulses. The impulses will be directed to specific locations in the cochlea based on pitch and loudness.

  Speech processors generally come in two styles. One is small enough to fit into the same headset or casing that contains the microphone and is worn behind the ear. The other style is about the size of a pager, which can be worn on a belt or carried in a pocket.
- Impulses from the speech processor are sent to a transmitter — sometimes called a transmitting coil. A

Transmitter

Receiver and stimulator

Cochlea

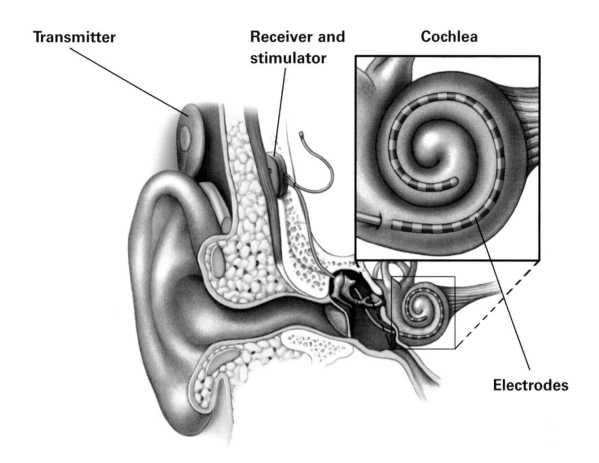

Electrodes

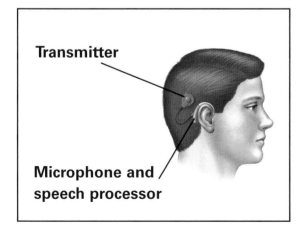

Transmitter

Microphone and speech processor

How an implant works

Cochlear implants use an external microphone and speech processor that you generally wear behind your ear. A transmitter sends radiofrequency signals to a surgically implanted electronic chip, the receiver-stimulator, that stimulates the auditory nerve with electrodes that have been threaded through the cochlea.

magnet holds the transmitter in place behind the ear, directly over a receiver-stimulator that's implanted beneath the scalp.

- The receiver-stimulator receives the impulses as radiofrequency waves from the transmitter. It relays the impulses as electronic signals through electrodes to the inner ear. The electrodes have been threaded directly into the cochlea on a bundle of tiny insulated wires.
- The electrodes stimulate the intact nerve fibers in the cochlea. This triggers the creation of electrical impulses. The impulses travel along the auditory nerve to the brain for processing and interpretation.

Although this multistage process seems quite complicated, the time it takes to happen is quite short. The length of time between when the microphone first picks up a sound and when the brain receives this information is just a few thousandths of a second. Any processing delay that occurs as a result of the cochlear implant isn't noticed by the user.

Research is currently under way to develop a completely implantable device — with no exterior component — in the not too distant future.

Implant candidates

Cochlear implants aren't alternatives to hearing aids. Rather, these devices best serve individuals for whom hearing aids will provide little or no benefit.

Candidates for a cochlear implant typically have severe to profound sensorineural hearing loss in both ears or have great difficulty understanding speech. However, the criteria for implantation have changed significantly over the years. Recently, individuals with some residual hearing remaining also are receiving implants.

Research is currently under way with new systems called hybrid implants. The devices are "hybrid" because they combine elements of electrical hearing (cochlear implant) and acoustical hearing (hearing aid). The implant portion stimulates only the parts of the cochlea responsible for mid- to high-frequency sounds. The hearing-aid portion, worn in the same ear, amplifies low-frequency sounds. This allows individuals with moderate to severe hearing loss and poor word recognition to improve their ability to understand speech.

Cochlear implants and the Deaf community

To the surprise of many people in the hearing world, many members of the Deaf community object to cochlear implants. For them, deafness isn't regarded as a disorder that needs to be treated or altered. They're often content within their unique culture, which includes a shared language (American Sign Language), social customs and lifestyle, and educational, economic, artistic and recreational institutions and organizations.

However, not all people who are deaf participate in Deaf culture. This has been a contentious issue for parents with children who are born deaf. In some situations, parents have received negative reactions if they choose a cochlear implant for their child rather than resources of the Deaf community.

Headway has been made in reconciling the two perspectives because many people recognize the value of being fluent in both worlds. Deaf and hearing-impaired people can continue to remain part of Deaf culture, but a cochlear implant allows them to have greater participation in hearing culture. However, research also indicates that the more heavily you rely on sign language, the less benefit you'll likely receive from a cochlear implant.

If you have profound hearing loss, you may find it helpful to talk to people with different viewpoints, such as those who use cochlear implants, those who use both sign and spoken language, and those who oppose implants. Such discussions can help you better understand the different perspectives and choose the best option for yourself.

The best age for implantation in children is debated, but most now receive implants between 1 and 3 years of age. In general, the younger a child is at the time of implantation, the less delay there will be in speech and language development — so long as appropriate therapy and education are provided following the procedure. Research indicates that getting a cochlear implant before age 3 will typically provide the best developmental outcomes.

Among adults, there's no upper age limit for implantation — even individuals in their 90s have received cochlear implants. Studies indicate that people over age 65 can experience excellent outcomes, providing significant benefits for both communication and awareness of the environment.

In addition to having hearing loss, candidates for a cochlear implant must:
- Have realistic expectations — a clear understanding of the benefits and limitations of the implant
- Be willing to commit to the pre-implant evaluations and post-surgical follow-up services
- Be motivated for the change, with the support of family and friends
- Be committed to being a part of the hearing world

The decision to receive an implant should be made only after talking to a cochlear implant audiologist and an experienced cochlear implant surgeon.

Contributing factors

Although thousands of people have received cochlear implants, no one can predict how much a given individual will benefit from the procedure. The results depend on several factors:

Duration of hearing loss

Adults and children who have experienced a relatively short period of severe to profound hearing loss will typically adapt to a cochlear implant more readily.

In contrast, individuals who have had profound hearing loss since birth or at a very young age typically have a harder time adjusting. In general, the shorter the duration of hearing loss, the better the outcome.

Also, individuals with some residual hearing tend to have better outcomes.

Auditory nerve fibers

People with a greater number of functioning nerve fibers in their cochlea may benefit more from a cochlear implant. No test can determine an exact number or location of functioning fibers, but imaging tests such as magnetic resonance imaging (MRI) and computerized tomography (CT) may provide valuable clues to the cochlear implant surgeon.

Sometimes, an electrical stimulation test can check if the auditory nerve will respond to small electrical signals.

Motivation

Much of the success of a cochlear implant depends on personal motivation and support. This commitment requires you to use the implant full time, maintain the equipment, keep follow-up appointments and take advantage of rehabilitation strategies.

Counseling is an important element of the implantation process. It can provide you with realistic expectations of the procedure. A cochlear implant is a tool, not a miracle cure. It will not restore normal hearing, but will give you the means to hear.

Benefits

According to reports from new users, hearing with a cochlear implant can range from "tinny" and "computer-like" to sounding almost normal. Generally, implant recipients notice the most improvement in their first year of using the device, but improvements can continue for many years after.

Generally, adult users are able to communicate more effectively and with less effort. Most recipients who are completely deaf are able to detect soft sounds, including low-level speech, and recognize many everyday noises.

Some individuals can receive greater benefits from their implants. Detecting voices in an adjoining room, talking on the telephone and enjoying music is within the realm of possibility.

For many children, a cochlear implant has an impact on their potential to develop spoken language. Many can receive most of their education without the use of sign language or other methods of speech representation.

In general, adults and children with cochlear implants can understand about 70 percent or more of full sentences and about 55 to 60 percent or more of single words that are spoken. When the speech occurs in a personal conversation or within a familiar context, the level of understanding is even better — especially if the conversation is direct and face to face.

The implant procedure

A cochlear implant program starts with a thorough evaluation of your hearing, which will guide many decisions made by you and your doctor. After the device has been implanted and activated, a series of follow-up sessions are necessary for speech and language training and rehabilitation.

Helping you through this process will be a team of specialists. Implant surgery is generally performed by an otolaryngologist, commonly known as an ear, nose and throat (ENT) doctor — although not all otolaryngologists perform the procedure. Other team members generally include an audiologist, speech-language pathologist and educational consultant.

Your doctor can refer you to a cochlear implant center for evaluation. Cochlear implant centers are located throughout the United States and in other countries. There are many issues to consider as you proceed with implantation, and the initial testing may help you.

Pre-implantation

A pre-implantation evaluation is undertaken by the implant team. The evaluation process can be stopped at any time that you or the implant team feel it's not appropriate to continue. The evaluation process includes the following tests:

Medical evaluation. The ENT doctor will examine the health and function of your ear (otological examination) to ensure that no active infection or any type of abnormality precludes the use of an implant. An internist may be asked to do a general physical examination to make sure you can safely undergo general anesthesia.

Imagery. The physician reviews X-rays, computerized tomography (CT) scans and magnetic resonance imaging (MRI) to study the auditory nerve and to see if the cochlea is suitable for inserting implant electrodes.

Costly procedure

The cost of getting a cochlear implant — including the pre-implant evaluation, surgery and hospital fees, medical personnel fees, implant hardware, and post-surgical fittings and training — is expensive. Some estimates range from $50,000 to $70,000. Unlike hearing aids, cochlear implants are covered by most private insurance plans, as well as Medicare and Medicaid programs. In some states, coverage is provided by children's special services, Tricare or state vocational rehabilitation agencies. Many patients receive the support of community or charitable organizations that hold special fundraisers, such as the Lions Club, Kiwanis, Sertoma and Jaycees.

Implant centers will likely have an insurance or reimbursement specialist who can help you determine the coverage provided by your health plan, and assist you with obtaining pre-authorization for coverage. It's important that you start the process early and allow your insurance company sufficient time to review your information before proceeding.

Audiological evaluation. The audiologist performs an extensive series of hearing tests to determine how well you can hear with and without appropriately adjusted hearing aids. A speech and language evaluation is performed for children to establish a baseline of their development prior to surgery. The baseline results are essential for monitoring progress in follow-up sessions after surgery.

Psychological evaluation. Some people may benefit from a psychological evaluation that may help them cope with lifestyle changes following the procedure. Many issues could affect their satisfaction with the implant.

If the results from these evaluations indicate that you're a good candidate for implantation, you can be scheduled for surgery. The surgeon will determine which ear would be best for the implant — usually it's the ear with the most severe hearing loss.

The surgeon may consider bilateral implants as your best option. It's becoming more common to implant devices in both ears of children and, in some cases, of adults as well. There's evidence that two implants help individuals identify the source of sounds and improve understanding of speech.

Before the surgery your implant team will discuss with you the benefits and limitations of a cochlear implant, care and use of the device, the surgery itself, and post-surgical follow-up. If you or a family member feels anxious during this process, feel free to ask questions and express your concerns.

Surgery

Cochlear implant surgery is performed under general anesthesia and lasts from two to four hours. Your doctor may do the procedure on an outpatient basis, or you may be asked to stay overnight at a hospital.

After anesthesia is administered, the surgeon makes an incision behind the ear and exposes the mastoid bone. A small depression is created in the bone, and the receiver-stimulator is placed in this depression.

A small portion of the mastoid bone is removed that allows access to the middle ear and the cochlea. A small hole is made in the cochlea, and tiny wires with the electrodes are inserted.

Electronic tests are performed to make sure the stimulator is functioning properly with the intact nerve fibers. Then the incision is closed.

When you wake up from anesthesia, you'll find a bulky bandage wrapped around your head. This will help reduce swelling around the incision.

You may experience some pain and nausea, but you can take medications for either form of discomfort. On the day of surgery, most people are able to get out of bed for short walks.

The day after surgery, the head bandage is removed. You may be given antibiotics to prevent infection, and will likely take prescription pain medication for the first three to four days.

Cochlear implants and meningitis

Cochlear implant recipients are at a slightly greater risk of bacterial meningitis, an infection in the lining of the brain's surface. Although the risk is considered very small, the incidence is taken seriously and has been thoroughly studied.

The cause of meningitis in implant recipients hasn't been firmly established but the design of earlier generations of implants is thought to be a factor. An implant, because it's a foreign body, may act as a breeding ground for infection — and the bacteria causing the infection may gain access to the brain via the pathway created by the implant electrodes. Some people may simply be more predisposed to meningitis due to abnormalities of the inner ear.

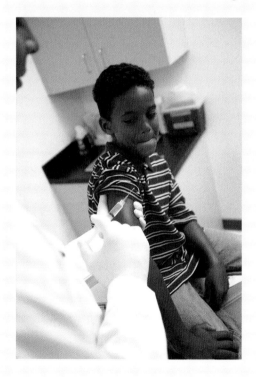

If you have a cochlear implant or are considering getting one, you should be vaccinated against the organisms that commonly cause bacterial meningitis. Pneumococcal vaccines often are recommended for children and for adults over age 65.

In the opinion of the FDA, the American Academy of Otolaryngology — Head and Neck Surgery and the League for the Hard of Hearing, the cochlear implant remains a safe, effective device that provides many benefits. Thousands of recipients have had cochlear implantation with no adverse side effects.

Complications of cochlear implant surgery are uncommon. Some people report a bitter or metallic taste or other differences in their sense of taste immediately after surgery, but this sensation eventually goes away.

Because the surgery involves your inner ear, your system of balance may be disrupted. This can cause dizziness or vertigo, which will usually improve over the first three to four days, followed by a period of mild unsteadiness for a few weeks. By gently increasing activity, even though you may be slightly dizzy, your balance should gradually return to normal.

The nerve controlling facial expressions runs through the surgical area. Rarely, the nerve may be weakened after surgery due to temporary swelling. You may notice that your smile isn't quite straight or you have trouble closing an eyelid. These signs can be treated with cortisone-type medication.

It takes up to four weeks after surgery for the incision to heal. Most recipients are able to resume normal activity within a few days to two weeks after surgery. Once the incision heals, the implant is noticeable on the outside only as a slight bump to the touch.

Activation

A cochlear implant is inactive while it's being implanted. Deciding the time to activate the device signals the next step in the implantation process.

It's preferable to wait at least one week or two before activating a cochlear implant. This allows time for the incision to heal, and for you to recover from the anesthesia. You'll then meet several times with the audiologist to complete the process of fitting the external components and programming (mapping) the speech processor.

For some adults, activation soon after surgery may be an option. This recourse is taken to decrease anxiety about the procedure. But at the same time, early activation may be somewhat uncomfortable and programming the device less precise.

At your initial session with the audiologist, the headset or speech processor containing the microphone is placed on your head. The processor is connected to the audiologist's computer and programming equipment. The transmitter also is positioned, held in place by a magnet that couples with the magnet in the implanted receiver.

One by one, the implanted electrodes embedded in your cochlea — each conveying a slightly different frequency or pitch — are turned on. You'll be asked to respond each time you hear a sound and to signal when the loudness of each sound is most comfortable.

The audiologist feeds this information into special computer software that programs your speech processor. The processor is set to certain levels of stimulation for each electrode, based on your responses.

After the programming is complete, the processor is disconnected from the audiologist's computer. Rechargeable or disposable batteries are inserted into the processor, and you're now able to take the system home.

Your audiologist will schedule more visits to fine-tune the speech processor. Repeated adjustments are necessary because it takes time for your auditory nerve to adapt to the signals from the electrodes and for your brain to interpret these signals.

Complete programming varies among different users and different implant systems. During the first year of use, the processor is reprogrammed often — you may have up to eight to 12 appointments. Fewer visits are required after that. Experienced users usually visit just once a year.

Adjusting to an implant

Everyone who receives a cochlear implant seems to have a different experience. Some users quickly appreciate sounds they haven't heard for many years. Other users need a gradual period of adjustment.

Typically, the sounds you first hear with a cochlear implant will seem unnatural. Often, speech will be unclear and hard to understand. With time, however, these sounds become more familiar as your brain relearns how to hear with the implant.

The process of adjustment is slow and can take anywhere from weeks to years. Users who haven't had a long period of hearing loss can often understand speech rather quickly without speech reading. Users who have never had hearing before often need a longer time to adjust to the sounds.

Care and handling

When you get a cochlear implant, members of your implant team will provide detailed instructions on how to take care of the external components of the system. The following tips may assist you:

- Always try to avoid environments of heavy moisture or extreme heat, or conditions that could cause breakage.
- On rainy or very humid days, keep a body-worn processor in a pouch or durable case that protects it from dampness. Watertight pouches are usually available at stores selling scubadiving equipment. If the speech processor is part of a headset, wear a hood when it's raining or snowing. Some newer headsets are manufactured as water-resistant.
- Remove external components before participating in water sports and activities that generate high levels of static electricity, such as using trampolines or plastic slides. Like other electronic devices, the speech processor can be damaged by static electricity.
- You can wear the implant while participating in most nonwater sports. While it doesn't require extraordinary precautions, it's always a good idea to wear protective headgear for activities such as bicycling, in-line skating, football and soccer. Avoid heading a soccer ball.
- Turn off the speech processor before changing batteries, replacing cords or plugging something into it.
- Don't store batteries in the refrigerator. Putting a cold battery in a processor may cause condensation problems.
- Keep the microphone and processor in an anti-humidity kit when not in use. This is sometimes called a dryer or dry-aid kit.

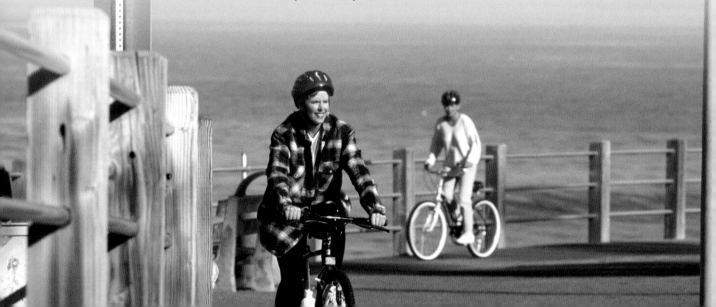

Learning to listen and make sense of the sounds requires your dedicated effort. It also requires consistent exposure to sound. Adjusting to a cochlear implant will be easier — and you'll gain greater benefit — if you wear the device full time.

Start out with easier listening situations, such as a conversation with one person in a quiet setting. With time, work up to more challenging situations, such as group conversations or listening in places where there's lots of background noise. Also practice listening to the radio and television.

Adult users can benefit from various support services. Working with an audiologist, speech-language pathologist or teacher of the hearing-impaired, you can practice identifying sounds, recognizing speech and using speech reading. Speech training can help you speak more clearly and with good voice quality.

Your training may include listening-only activities and practice with a telephone. You may be given instructions on how to continue auditory training at home. Many Web-based programs are available over the Internet for free or at a marginal cost that can help.

Rehabilitation training and education are essential for children who receive a cochlear implant. Without such training and education, a child will obtain only partial benefit from the device. Your child must learn to associate meanings to all of the new, unfamiliar sounds. They must be taught to understand the sounds and integrate them into language.

Speech-language pathologists, educators and family members can help reinforce the skills that your child is learning. The process takes time, dedication and a lot of hard work. But throughout childhood, training will usually continue to improve performance.

Your audiologist or speech-language pathologist can provide you with other strategies to improve communication and handle difficult listening situations (see also Chapter 6).

Stay positive

Individual personality and many psychological factors can have strong impacts on your level of satisfaction with a cochlear implant. For example, whether you're a pessimist or an optimist, whether you carry moderate or high expectations of the procedure, and whether you have a weak or strong support network can influence your outcome with the implant.

You can boost your chances of success with a positive attitude. A person who's inflexible and pessimistic may look for — and find — all the wrong things about an implant, regardless of how well it functions.

In contrast, an optimistic person will keep the adjustment period in perspective and focus on positive improvements that can be made. If you expect to hear speech clearly in the first days after your implant is programmed, you'll likely be disappointed.

A good support system is also very important. Let your family and friends know how they can help you succeed with an implant. You can also talk to your audiologist about any problems you're having as you adjust. At least once a year, return for a checkup at the cochlear implant center or clinic where you had your surgery.

Staying positive won't prevent you from experiencing a wide range of emotions about the implant, both posi-tive and negative. Having the procedure triggers many emotions — and no one's reaction is the same. Whatever your experience, give yourself time to adjust and become used to hearing again. Most people adapt in their own way in their own time.

Other options to communicate better

Hearing aids and cochlear implants are valuable tools if you have a hearing impairment. But other options, including special listening devices, wireless technology and even your cell phone, can help you in many challenging situations.

These technologies can resolve common problems you face every day and make your life easier and safer — by alerting you to a doorbell ring, by allowing you to listen to television at a reasonable volume and converse on the telephone, and by giving you the freedom to participate in different kinds of public events and activities.

The communication technologies don't replace hearing aids or cochlear implants. Rather they support these devices and enhance your hearing in difficult listening environments — such as noisy restaurants or lecture halls where sound reverberates. They allow you to lead a more independent and flexible lifestyle.

Special devices are useful for the times when you aren't wearing your hearing aids, such as when you're in bed or in the shower. They can alert you to sounds you need to be aware of, such as an alarm clock, smoke alarm or security alarm.

A variety of devices and services are available for you to use, both at home and in public places, including offices, restaurants, hospitals, places of worship, hotels, theaters, airports, trains, buses, libraries and courtrooms.

Under the Americans With Disabilities Act (ADA) and other federal legislation, public places are required to make reasonable accommodation for people who are deaf or hearing impaired. What is meant by "reasonable" may vary according to the type of establishment and the circumstances but may include different types of assistive listening devices, captioning services and alerting technology.

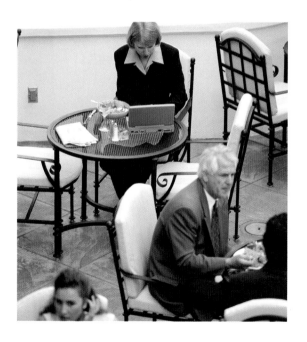

Assistive listening devices

A sudden, loud noise measuring 140 decibels (dB) or more, or a noise exceeding 85 dB that's sustained over an eight-hour period, is considered to be hazardous to your hearing.

Many situations in daily life at more tolerable noise levels nevertheless can disrupt your ability to hear and to function effectively. Three factors are often involved, either alone or in combination, to cause the problem.

Noise. The hum of an air ventilation system, traffic sounds or the scraping of chairs on the floor may prevent you from understanding what's being said.

Reverberation. Confined areas that have many hard surfaces, concrete block walls or uncarpeted floors are likely to be reverberant — they easily echo sounds. The surfaces reflect sound waves multiple times so that the sound persists, even after the sound source is cut off.

Distance. The farther away you are from a speaker — or the farther off to the side you are — the harder it can be to hear. The best distance for hearing speech is between three and six feet.

Even with the help of hearing aids, these factors in certain environments will create severe acoustic difficulties. The environments include:

- Places with a lot of commotion and background noise, such as restaurants, cafeterias, lobbies, malls, subways and airports. An office can be a noisy place with the sound of foot traffic, conversation, manufacturing equipment, printers, copiers, telephones and radio.
- Situations where several people are talking at once, such as parties and social gatherings.
- Large rooms and facilities where a speaker may be far away, such as worship halls, classrooms, theaters and stadiums.
- Locations that are highly reverberant and sound waves echo, such as classrooms, hallways, basements, open offices, worship halls, arenas and warehouses.
- Situations where a steady, constant background noise is created by a fan, air conditioner, traffic or wind. This type of noise includes travel noise from highways or rails when you're riding in a car or train.

- Outdoor activities where sound waves are dispersed, such as sporting events, festivals, parades, picnics and barbecues.
- Telephone conversations, especially when the connection isn't clear. The fact that you can't rely on visual cues affects your understanding.

Many of these environments are difficult, if not impossible, to avoid and hard to plan for. Yet circumstances often require you to participate in them as you go about your daily life. Your ability to function effectively can benefit greatly from specialized technology developed specifically for these challenging environments.

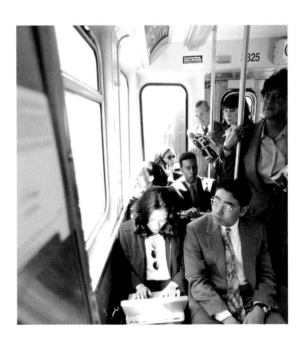

Assistive listening devices (ALDs) are designed to improve your ability to hear in situations where conventional hearing aids aren't sufficient. ALDs are useful for many social, educational, and entertainment activities, as well as for personal use at home.

These devices can help you in noisy rooms and in group conversations. They make it easier to use a telephone. In addition, ALDs may be used in one-on-one conversations with a friend and for listening to television or radio while you're relaxing alone.

Several ALDs are designed for use in large rooms, where people with hearing loss may have trouble understanding a distant speaker at a podium or on a stage. Frequently, in these settings listeners face problems not only because of distance from the speaker but also because of reverberation and background noise.

In classrooms, teachers often move from side to side or turn away from the class, so the volume of their speech fluctuates. In these situations, asking the teacher to talk louder may not solve your problems. Turning up the volume increases audibility but it may not make speech more intelligible.

ALDs work by making the sound or signal you want to hear stand out from noise you don't want or need to hear. The signal might be a faraway voice coming over a static-filled telephone line, or a companion's voice that gets lost in the clatter of a noisy restaurant.

Although ALDs can usually amplify sounds, their primary purpose isn't to make sounds louder. Rather, they place a microphone close to the source of the sound you want to hear so that sound is clearer and louder than other sounds in your environment.

ALD systems are equipped with different microphones, headphones and other features, but all systems are based on two components: a transmitter and a receiver.

The transmitter, located close to the person speaking, picks up the sounds and converts them to signals, then broadcasts the signals. Often, there's a direct hookup to a microphone.

The receiver, located close to a listener, picks up the signals and introduces them to the listener's ears. Receivers carried by different individuals in the same audience can pick up the same signal from a single transmitter.

Some ALDs are designed for use with hearing aids or cochlear implants, and others are used alone. Many that are used with hearing aids require that the hearing aid have a feature such as a telecoil (t-coil), telephone switch or hookup (port) for direct audio input.

Telephonic devices

Using the telephone can be a special challenge. For one thing, a conventional telephone doesn't amplify sound loud enough for individuals with hearing loss. For another thing, the listeners can't rely on visual cues to help their understanding.

One of the most common and useful ALDs is a telephone amplifier, which may be used with a cell phone or with a wired, cordless or digital phone. The amplifier allows a user to adjust the volume of incoming calls so that even soft voices can be heard. It also allows a person with no hearing loss to easily use the device as well.

An amplifier may be installed in the telephone body or in the handset when

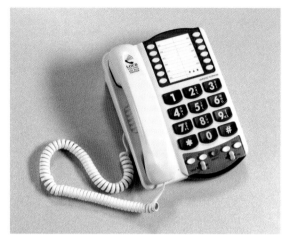

Amplified telephone

A decal on the phone receiver indicates that this phone can amplify a speaker's voice. The controls at the bottom of the phone body allow you to adjust the volume to your preference.

the mouthpiece, receiver and buttons are included as one unit. Many new telephones come directly from the manufacturer with a built-in amplifier. An amplifier also may be added as an in-line unit between the telephone and wall jack.

Amplifier handsets may be installed in some public telephones, particularly at airports, train stations, museums and hotel lobbies. A special telephone access sign on the receiver will identify whether the service is available.

Portable, snap-on amplifiers are small, battery-operated devices that can be carried with you in a purse or brief-case. When you're in situations where it's unlikely that you'll find a phone with an amplifier handset, you can slip the device over the receiver of most telephones. These portable amplifiers are especially helpful when you're traveling and on the run.

Telephone adapters are also portable devices that work with the telecoil in your hearing aids or cochlear implants. The adapter doesn't amplify sound but instead generates an electromagnetic field in response to sound waves. This allows the telecoil to pick up the sound directly. An adapter may work with some phones that aren't compatible with portable amplifiers.

Using your hearing aid's telecoil

Many behind-the-ear and in-the-ear hearing aids are equipped with a telecoil (t-coil). The telecoil is helpful for listening on the telephone. Normally, a hearing aid is sensitive to all sound waves. But when you turn on the telecoil, the aid amplifies only electromagnetic waves from the telephone's receiver. This means that the telephone signal is transmitted directly into the hearing aid without any other noise being amplified.

Most phones are compatible with hearing aids, but when you buy a phone, be sure to ask about hearing aid compatibility. If the salesperson doesn't know, try out the phone before buying it. The telecoil can also be used with FM systems (see page 194) and induction loop systems (see page 198).

Having a hearing aid with a telecoil broadens your communication options. If your hearing aid has a telecoil and you aren't sure how to use it, consult your audiologist or hearing aid dealer for training.

Buying ALDs and other communication aids

Many assistive listening devices (ALDs) are provided free of charge in public places. If you're planning to buy an ALD or another form of communication aid for personal use, discuss the different options with your audiologist. Various devices may be on display at a local audiological center or speech, language and hearing center, university, or community agency. Web sites also offer a wide selection of products with in-depth information.

These devices vary in price, so it's wise to comparison shop and work with someone who's knowledgeable of the technology. Check the warranty before you buy — some products come with as much as a five-year warranty. The staff who dispense ALDs should provide you with training, including how to check and recharge batteries.

Many newer phones don't function with either a telecoil or portable amplifier. Always check beforehand to learn whether your phone is compatible.

Some telephones have special ringers that produce either an extra-loud ring or variable rings. Call indicators use a flashing light to inform you of incoming calls. Speaker phones can be useful in certain situations because they allow a person with hearing loss to listen with both ears.

Telecommunication relay service

People with severely limited hearing or no hearing at all can't use a standard telephone, even with an amplifier or adapter. They can still communicate over phone lines, however, by using a telecommunication relay service (TRS).

TRS is a public service that comes at no cost to its users — the Americans With Disabilities Act requires U.S. telephone

Telephones for hearing impairment

If you have severe or profound hearing loss, using text-to-voice or captioned forms of TRS with a communications assistant requires that you have a special telephone with a display screen for text.

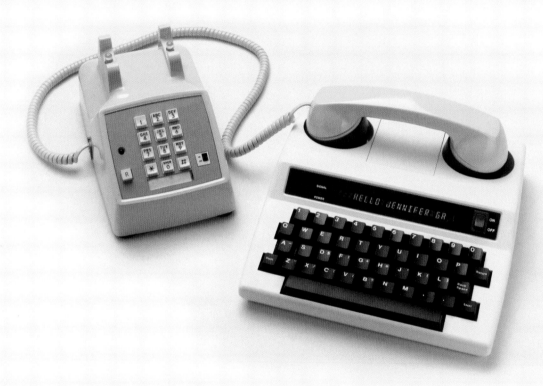

Text telephone. A telecommunication device for the deaf (TDD) is a telephone hooked up to a keyboard. It was formerly called a teletypewriter (TTY). If you have hearing loss, you type what you want to say, and the communications assistant relays the message verbally. A spoken response appears, via the communications assistant, as text on your screen.

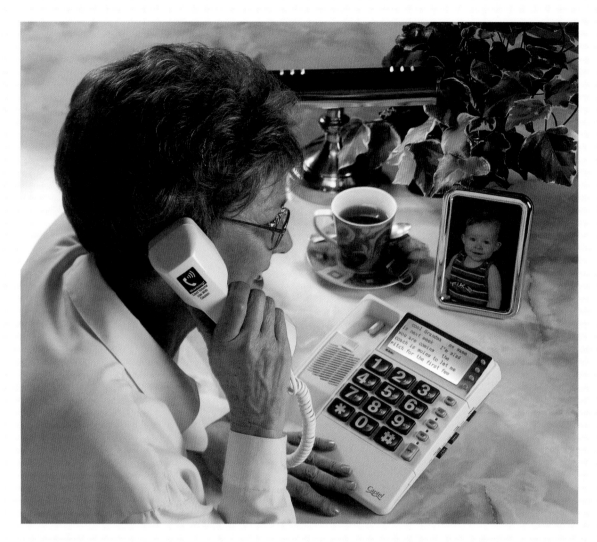

Captioned telephone. This device allows you to hear the caller's voice and simultaneously see what's being said. The captions entered by a communications assistant appear on your telephone's text screen. You place a call in the same way that you would dial on a standard telephone, and you're automatically connected to the captioning service.

companies to provide the service free throughout the country. The phone companies are compensated with either state or federal funds.

Using TRS requires an individual with hearing loss to have a special phone equipped with a keyboard and text display monitor — a text telephone — or a captioned telephone (see pages 188-189). Certain types of relay services also function with a home computer.

TRS provides real-time communication by adding a third-party operator, called a communications assistant (CA), into your phone conversation. The CAs are on call 24 hours a day at TRS relay centers located throughout the country.

You provide the CA with the telephone number to be called, either by speaking it into the handset or by typing and sending it via the keyboard. The CA places the call and then relays spoken and written messages back and forth between you and your correspondent.

The CA quickly converts spoken or written words into either text or voice. CAs are trained to be unobtrusive and to relay your conversations exactly as they're received. All calls through TRS are strictly confidential.

The telecommunications relay service is easy to use. Anyone can initiate a call by dialing 711 — the number that the federal government has reserved for access to TRS. Callers pay only the normal cost of a phone call.

There are several forms of TRS to consider, depending on your hearing loss and your personal preference:

Text-to-voice. This is the standard method described above, with a CA serving as an intermediary between the spoken and written portions of the phone conversation. The CA manually types the written text.

A voice-carry-over (VCO) option allows a person with hearing loss to speak directly to the other person instead of corresponding through a CA. Similarly, with hearing-carry-over (HCO) a person with speech impairment can still hear the other party's voice and then relay a typed response through the CA.

Captioned service. This form of TRS uses voice recognition technology to convert the CA's spoken voice into written text. The captions are transmitted directly to a text display screen on your telephone.

Internet protocol (IP) relay service. With this Internet-based form of TRS, a call goes from your computer to an IP relay center, which is usually accessed from a Web page. The CA relays your message via spoken voice over the regular telephone network.

You're not required to have a text or captioned telephone to use this service. A computer or any other Web-enabled device such as a cell phone will do. The service connects directly to many forms of instant messaging and wireless text messaging programs.

IP captioned telephone service combines the Internet-based system with a captioned telephone display. You speak directly to the called party and can listen to the response. At the same time, the CA repeats what's being said and speech recognition technology allows you to see the words almost instantaneously on your computer display.

Video relay service (VRS). Another Internet-based form of TRS is a bridge between individuals using sign language and individuals using spoken English. A CA communicates with the sign language user via a computer monitor and video equipment. Not all state TRS programs offer this service.

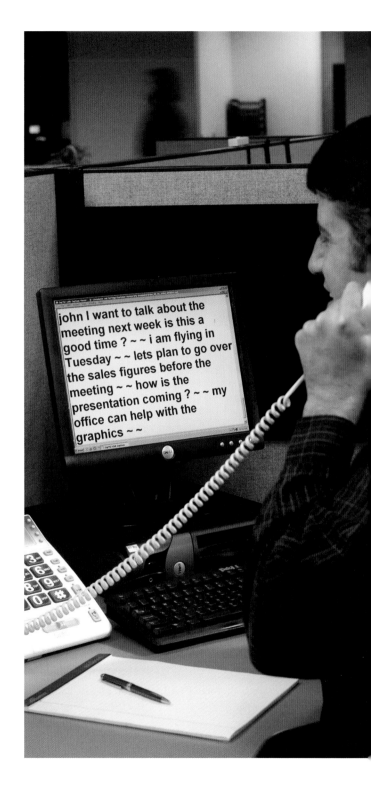

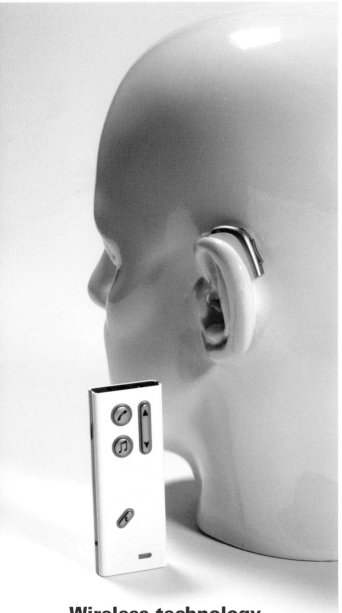

Wireless technology

The push of a button on this remote connects your hearing aid to the telephone or allows you to listen to music from your portable music player without any direct hookup.

Multipurpose communication devices

Advances in computer hardware and electronics continue to create smaller and more adaptable devices. This helps make many communication aids more portable, flexible and convenient.

Single devices have been developed that combine multiple functions. For example, a device that may look and function as a hearing aid — when needed — is also capable of other functions, serving as your wireless telephone with access to the Internet, voice mail and more.

Wireless technology takes these developments a step further. Wireless networks use low-power radio waves to link computers and other devices together — no wires or cable hookups are required for them to communicate. Generally, the different units must be located close together.

Bluetooth technology can connect as many as eight different devices together at the same time. That means — so long as all the devices are Bluetooth-enabled — your hearing aid, computer, telephone and music player can be interacting simultaneously.

Text messaging

Cell phones have become exceedingly popular communication tools worldwide. People use these portable, easy-to-use devices not only for phone calls but for taking pictures, accessing the Internet, and playing music and games as well.

Text messaging is another popular use of cell phones. Using the phone keypad as a keyboard, you can type text messages into your phone — generally up to 160 characters — and send them to one or more other phones. This means of communication is known as short message service (SMS).

SMS is a valuable new tool for people with moderate to profound hearing loss, particularly because use is so quick and simple. You're able to communicate just about anywhere with many more people, and you're not tied to a TTD or computer. Furthermore, cell phones have become so pervasive in society that they call little attention to the fact that you have hearing loss.

A drawback is that cell phones can cause interference with hearing aids — typically a buzzing sound. To make cell

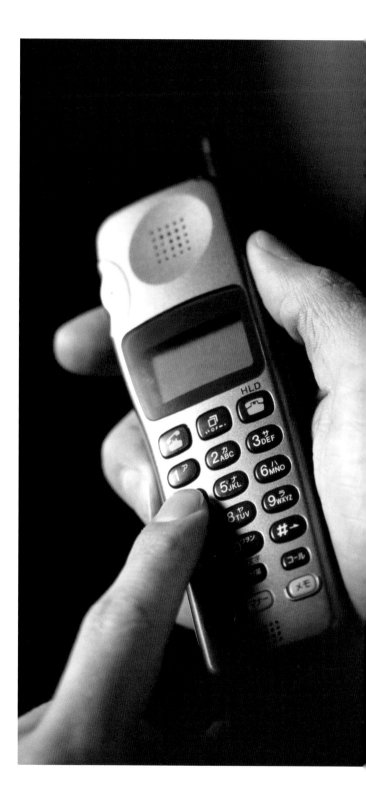

phones more accessible, the Federal Communications Commission (FCC) has approved standards for the use of digital wireless devices with hearing aids in the Hearing Aid Compatibility (HAC) Act.

A HAC-compliant cell phone will be marked with M or T ratings. The *M* refers to phone use when the hearing aid is set to microphone. The *T* refers to phone use when the hearing aid is set to telecoil.

For best results and less interference, your cell phone should have a rating of M3 or M4 and T3 or T4. If these ratings are not marked on the package, inquire with your service provider or the device manufacturer.

Assistive listening systems

Assistive listening systems improve the sound quality and volume of public address systems for people with hearing loss. One of three systems generally will be installed in public places for this purpose: FM, infrared and induction loop.

FM systems

At public-speaking events, you may be seated at some distance away and not directly in front of the speaker. The amplification system is poor quality, and the audience members are moving about and talking among themselves. You may still be able to hear the speaker clearly with the help of special listening systems, such as an FM system.

You may be familiar with the letters *FM* (frequency modulation) from tuning your radio to a specific frequency in order to hear your favorite music or talk show. FM listening systems transmit sounds via radio waves, just like a miniature radio station. They operate on special radiofrequencies assigned by the FCC. FM systems are commonly installed in locations where large audiences gather, such as auditoriums, convention centers, places of worship, museums and theaters.

With FM systems, sounds are broadcast by a wireless radio transmitter to small, portable receivers tuned to the correct FM frequency. The receivers are earphones worn by listeners in the audience. The transmitter can broadcast anything from a microphone, radio, television or stereo.

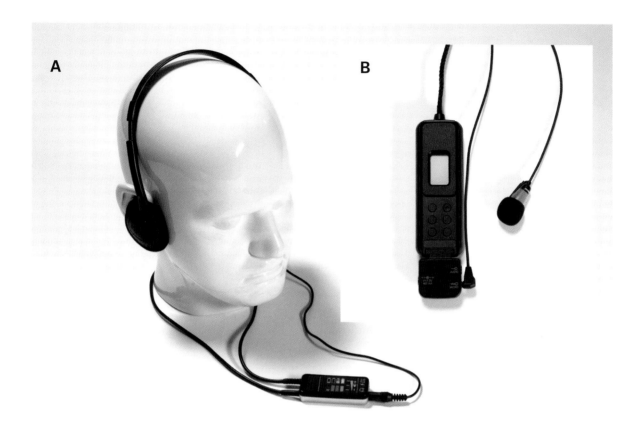

A

B

FM systems

In a setting with a large audience, such as a classroom, an FM system with a transmitter and microphone (B) allows speakers to send their voices directly to you through a receiver that you wear with headphones (A) or hearing aids.

FM systems also can be used with hearing aids or cochlear implants equipped with a telecoil or audio input. To use the telecoil, you wear a looped cord of wire that converts the FM signal into electromagnetic waves that are picked up by your telecoil.

If you don't have a telecoil, you can link to the FM system using a small adapter called a boot. All cochlear implants and several styles of behind-the-ear hearing aids are manufactured in the United States equipped to receive FM signals.

Assisted listening systems

FM system

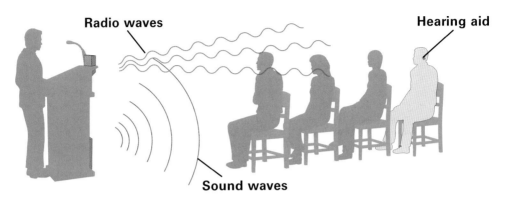

Radio waves

Hearing aid

Sound waves

Infrared system

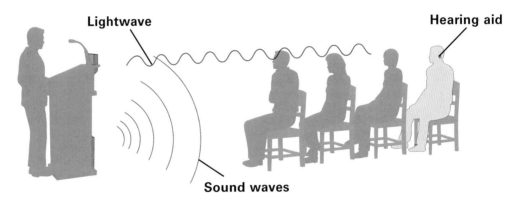

Lightwave

Hearing aid

Sound waves

Induction loop system

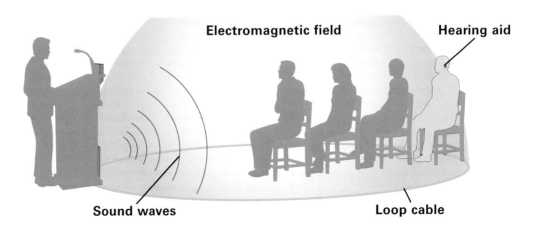

Electromagnetic field

Hearing aid

Sound waves

Loop cable

Personal FM systems can be used for one-on-one communication. Composed of a small, portable microphone, receiver and amplifier, they're useful for private conversations in difficult hearing environments such as noisy restaurants or highly reverberant auditoriums. As long as you're tuned to the correct frequency, you can use personal systems while you're walking or in a car, and you can use them to listen to television and radio stations.

A growing number of public buildings, government facilities and business offices are equipped with FM systems to accommodate hearing-impaired visitors. Many schools also are using FM technology to assist students with hearing impairment.

Infrared systems

Radio waves aren't the only medium available to carry sound in assistive listening systems. Infrared systems transmit sound via lightwaves to receivers worn by hearing-impaired listeners.

Like FM systems, infrared systems are used in locations where hearing is difficult or large groups of people gather. Infrared technology is also commonly available for TV viewing at home.

When this system is used in a large auditorium, an infrared light emitter is plugged into an existing public-address system or sound system. The infrared lightwaves transmit speech or music to receivers worn by members of the audience. The receiver may be a headphone that introduces sound directly to the ear. Or the receiver can be used with a hearing aid or cochlear implant equipped with a telecoil.

Using an infrared system with a television allows you to set the TV at a volume that's lower and more comfortable for other listeners. The infrared transmitter sends the TV signal to a personal receiver, which you can adjust to as loud a volume as you need. But your adjustments don't affect the volume level heard by others in the room.

Unlike an FM system, an infrared receiver must be in the transmitter's direct line of broadcast in order to function well. Sunlight can interfere with the signal, so these systems aren't a good choice for outdoor use.

In contrast, because infrared lightwaves are broadcast along a confined path and not emitted in all directions, infrared systems provide more privacy than FM systems do. Infrared systems

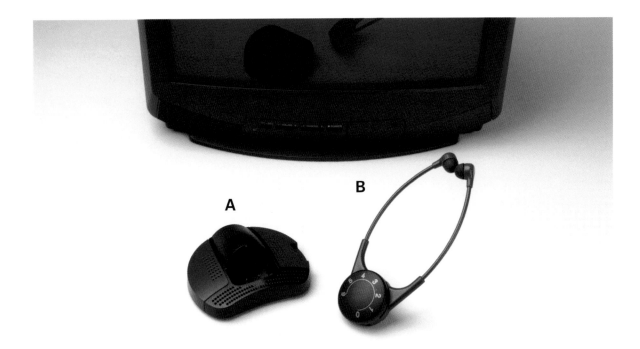

Infrared systems

Infrared systems send sounds, for example from a television program, directly to you from a unit that sits on the television (A). A lightweight headset that you wear (B) lets you adjust the device to a volume that you need for hearing while keeping the TV at a volume that's comfortable for others.

are often used in courtrooms and government offices and during live performances in theaters and auditoriums.

Induction loop systems

Induction loop systems, also called audio loop systems, generally are not used as commonly as FM systems or infrared systems. Induction loop systems transmit sounds using an electromagnetic field created by a loop of wire installed around the listening area. An amplifier and microphone transmit sound via an electric current that flows through the loop. Hearing aids and cochlear implants equipped with telecoils can receive these signals. Separate receivers can be provided to people who don't have the telecoil feature.

Induction loop systems can be permanently installed in the floors of large auditoriums or chambers. Portable, impermanent loop systems may be set up as needed. Reception with these systems is susceptible to electrical interference. Also, they're not as flexible for personal use as FM systems and infrared systems are.

Captioning

Until the early 1970s, many people with hearing loss weren't able to fully enjoy one of America's favorite pastimes — watching television. In 1972, for the first time, a national TV program — Julia Child's cooking show, "The French Chef" — was broadcast with captions that reflected the audio portion of the show.

Since that broadcast, captions have opened the world of television to people who are deaf or hearing impaired. Hundreds of hours of entertainment, news, public affairs and sports programming are captioned each week on network, public and cable TV.

Similar to movie subtitles, television captions display dialogue as printed

International symbols

When these symbols appear in public buildings, it means services have been installed for individuals with hearing loss.

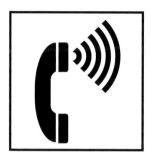

Amplified telephone

Text telephone

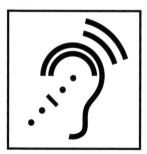

Assistive listening system

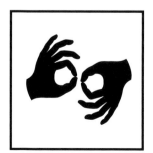

Sign language

words on the screen. Unlike subtitles, captions also indicate sounds such as noise, music and laughter. The text is carefully positioned on the screen to identify who is speaking. Captions are encoded as data within the television signal, ready for immediate broadcast.

Captions may be displayed as open or closed. Open captions appear on all TV screens and can be viewed without a special decoder. Closed captions aren't visible on a standard screen. To display the captions, you need a television with a built-in decoder or an added decoder that sits on top of the set.

With either form of decoder, you turn the captions on or off with the touch of a button on the remote. Since 1993, all television sets with screens 13 inches or larger sold in the United States have built-in decoder circuitry. Because of the widespread availability of closed captioning, open captions are rarely used.

You can tell if a specific program is closed captioned when the letters CC appear on the screen, often within a television-shaped symbol. Another symbol shows a small TV screen with a tail at the bottom.

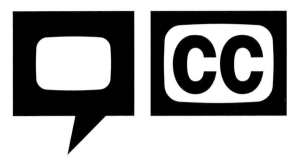

Closed caption symbols

Either of these symbols indicate that a television program is closed captioned.

Other uses of captioning

Captioning is included on many movies that are for sale or rent on DVD and VHS tape. It's also featured on many educational and training films.

Captioning is provided for many live events, such as musical and theater performances, lectures, government proceedings, meetings and conferences. Museums and science centers may use captioning in their self-produced films, demonstrations and shows.

Some movie theaters offer a captioning system called Rear Window captioning. An adjustable transparent plastic panel attaches to the viewer's seat and reflects captions displayed on a panel positioned at the back of the theater.

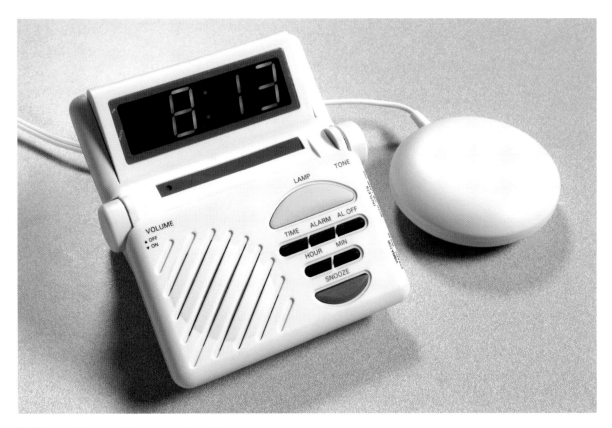

Vibrating alarm clock

This alarm clock can employ any or all of three options to wake you: a loud sound, a flashing light and a vibrating attachment that can be placed under your pillow to gently shake you.

Alerting devices

Assistive technology can alert you to many special sounds in your environment. Awareness of these sounds is important for your safety and to maintain your independent lifestyle. Sounds that can be signaled include a telephone ring, alarm clock buzz, kitchen timer beep, doorbell chime, a knock at the door, the cry of a baby, and the peal of a smoke alarm or security alarm.

Alerting devices may use one or more of three types of signal to inform you of the sound — an amplified sound, a flashing light or a vibration.

For example, an alarm clock can be wired with a vibrating attachment that's placed under your pillow. At the selected hour, you're gently shaken awake. Another option is an attachment with a flashing light that's plugged into your regular alarm clock.

Devices such as a vibrating pager or wristwatch can alert you in response to a paging system or time setting.

Alerting systems may be simple or complex. Some multipurpose alarms can use a code to indicate different sounds — for example, a telephone ring might be one light flash, the doorbell three flashes and the smoke alarm a series of on-off flashes. Some systems can be wired for use in several rooms or for transferring from room to room.

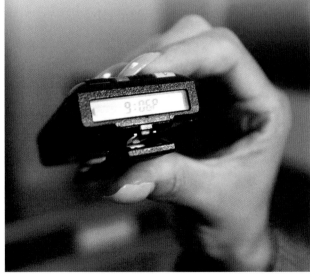

Special alerting devices can be used in your vehicle. A siren alert can let you know when an emergency vehicle is approaching. A blinker buddy tells you that the turn signal is on with a flashing light and a sound that gets louder the longer the signal remains on.

On the horizon

It wasn't that long ago that hearing aids were just about the only communication aid available for people with hearing loss. Now, advances in computer engineering and miniaturization are creating new technology and applications and bringing about major improvements to existing devices. Researchers continue to search for new ways to improve people's lives.

Speech recognition systems

One area of research and development is speech recognition, also referred to as voice recognition. Speech recognition allows you to control a computer by speaking to it rather than using a keyboard and mouse. When you speak, your commands appear as text on the computer screen.

The first speech recognition machine was created in 1950. But in 1997, continuous-speech-recognition software became commercially available — which means the machine is able to interpret a voice at a normal conversational rate. These systems are relatively inexpensive and easy to use.

Speech recognition systems can be very useful for someone with hearing impairment. They allow you to capture voices with a microphone and convert what's being said into a visual display on a screen.

Learning to use the software, however, requires special training and patience. You prepare by entering specialized words into the program and training the system to recognize voice patterns.

The technology is still not able to handle tricky listening environments. For example, you can't walk into a noisy party, point the microphone in the direction of a speaker and instantly read his or her words on a screen.

The technology is also being explored as a way to help people who rely primarily on speech reading to communicate. As someone speaks, a computer uses speech recognition and other software to create a sequence of visual cues — hand shapes — that help a speech reader distinguish between different speech elements that look similar when spoken. With video equipment, the cues are superimposed over an image of the speaker's face, allowing the speech reader to follow real-time conversation more easily.

Visual communication systems

Visual communication technology has great potential for people with hearing loss, especially those who use sign language as their primary means of communication. This system typically involves the use of video and computer equipment to allow people to communicate in sign language over the phone lines or the Internet.

One computer program under development provides real-time translation of spoken or written English into sign language. The hearing party's words are captured by a microphone or inputted as text and displayed on the recipient's computer screen as a signing figure. Another system provides sign language by way of a computer that's fitted with a digital camera and on-call interpreters.

Many options

Many people with hearing loss aren't aware of the numerous options in technology and computer software that can make communication easier. Assistive listening devices and other communication aids can make a significant difference in easing the daily problems caused by hearing loss. It's worthwhile to explore these options.

Of course, choosing among this ever-changing technology and knowing what might work best for you can be confusing at first. It's all too easy to be overawed or seduced by the gadgetry. If you're not sure where to start, talk to a hearing health professional, such as your audiologist or ENT doctor.

Chapter 10

Problems with balance

T he word *dizzy* is used to describe a variety of sensations — an illusion of motion, lightheadedness, weakness, loss of balance, faintness, wooziness and unsteadiness on your feet. You may feel that your surroundings are spinning around you — a condition commonly called vertigo. Imbalance occurs when you have to support yourself or hold on to something in order to maintain your balance.

There are many causes of dizziness, disrupting the complex system of balance in your body. A critical element of this system is the vestibular labyrinth that, together with the cochlea, is con-

tained in your inner ear. That explains why certain disorders of the inner ear produce both hearing loss and dizziness as symptoms.

Dizziness is the third most common reason why people over age 65 visit their doctor. Aging increases your risk of certain conditions that cause dizziness but especially imbalance.

Although it may be temporarily disabling, dizziness rarely signals a serious, life-threatening situation. Doctors often can determine the cause of dizziness, and for most people the signs and symptoms last a short time. Even when no cause is found or the dizziness persists, your doctor can prescribe treatments that usually ease symptoms to a manageable level.

Keeping yourself balanced

Your system of balance allows you to remain upright as you walk and move around or change position, for example, from a sitting to standing position. The system helps keep your vision focused and clear while your head is turning. Good balance also keeps you aware of the position of your head in relation to the ground.

To maintain your balance, your brain must coordinate sensory information coming from your eyes, inner ear, the bottoms of your feet, and major joints such as the ankles, knees and neck. Then the brain signals the muscles throughout your body on how to react and maintain your position.

This same information helps form your perceptions of how you're oriented in space, what direction you're moving in and how fast you're moving.

Your eyes. No matter what position you're in — sitting, standing or lying down, moving upright or crouched — visual signals help you determine where your body is in space. When light hits the photosensitive cells of your retina, it generates electrical impulses that are communicated to the brain through the optic nerve.

Your brain interprets these signals as images. The brain uses the images to calculate, for example, how far your chair seat is above the ground or how far away a car is that's moving in front of you, or how fast you're moving relative to someone walking beside you.

Your nervous system. Millions of nerve cells (neurons) are located in your skin, muscles and joints. When touch, pressure and movement stimulate these cells, they send electrical impulses to your brain about what your body is doing — for example, whether it's lying down on a soft mattress or climbing up a stepladder.

Information about the movement of your neck and your ankles is particularly important for balance because it indicates to your brain which way your head is turned and how steady you are on the ground.

Your system of balance

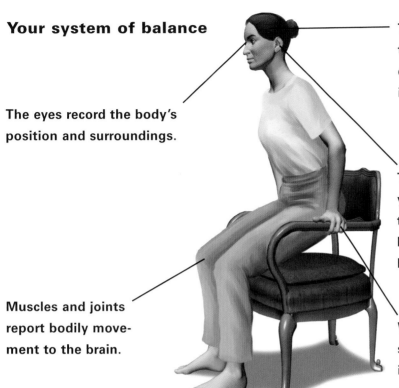

The eyes record the body's position and surroundings.

The brain relays information to and from the eyes, muscles and joints, skin and inner ear.

The inner ear contains both your primary hearing structure (cochlea) and primary balance structure (vestibular labyrinth).

Muscles and joints report bodily movement to the brain.

When you touch things, sensors in your skin give you information about your environment.

Your vestibular labyrinth. The vestibular labyrinth is your primary balance organ. The brain uses this organ in your inner ear to determine where your head is relative to gravitational space, and whether your head or body is changing its position in space.

Although you may not be as aware of the vestibular labyrinth as you are of your eyes, your brain relies on its input for balance — particularly when information from the eyes, joints or bottoms of your feet is in some way disrupted.

Problems with dizziness and balance can arise anywhere within this complex, interconnected sensory system. In order for you to be able to maintain your balance across a full range of daily activities, at least two of the three elements — the eyes, musculoskeletal nerves and vestibular labyrinth — must be working well.

For example, closing your eyes in the shower while washing your hair doesn't mean you'll lose your balance. That's because signals from your inner

Your vestibular system at work

The vestibular labyrinth is located just behind the cochlea in your inner ear. It consists of three fluid-filled loops called the semicircular canals. The base of each canal widens into a section known as the ampulla, which holds the hair cells that keep your brain informed of the rotational or turning motions of your head.

The three semicircular canals are connected to the central structure of the vestibular labyrinth called the vestibule. Within the vestibule are two chambers called the utricle and the saccule. The utricle is the upper chamber connecting all three semicircular canals. The saccule is the lower chamber. These chambers help monitor the position of your head in relation to up and down motion and forward and backward motion, such as when you ride in an elevator or a car.

Both the utricle and the saccule contain a patch of sensory hair cells embedded in a gel-like substance. These patches contain tiny particles called otoconia (o-toe-KOE-nee-uh). When you go up in an elevator, the otoconia in the saccule — responsible for detecting vertical movement — are pulled down by gravity. When you move forward in a car, the otoconia in the utricle — responsible for detecting horizontal movement — are pulled backward.

With either action, the otoconia pull the gel-like substance with them. The gel, in turn, stimulates the embedded hair cells, triggering electrical impulses that are sent along the nerve pathways to your brain with information about your vertical and horizontal movements. In similar fashion, impulses from your semicircular canals also provide information about angular changes in the position of your head, such as tilting to the left or right.

Your brain responds to these impulses, regardless of what you're doing, by signaling your eyes to move in the opposite direction of your head, keeping the image you're looking at focused on the retina. Your brain also signals the skeletal muscles to react quickly to help you keep your body balanced.

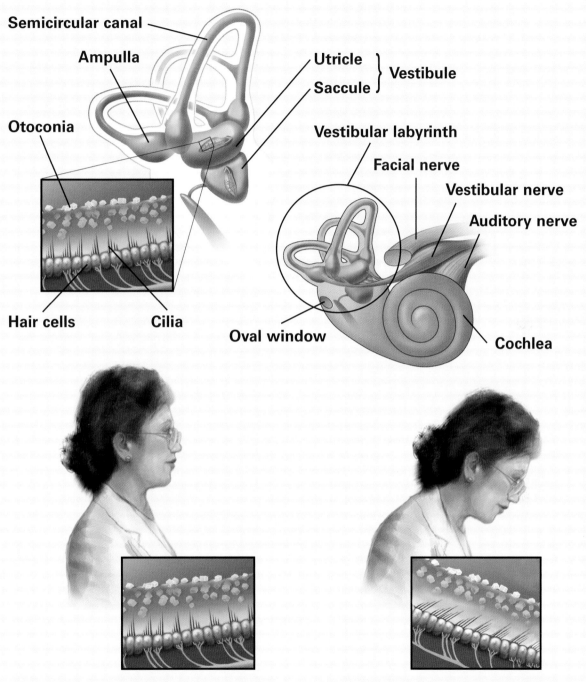

Semicircular canal

Ampulla

Otoconia

Hair cells   Cilia

Utricle
Saccule } Vestibule

Vestibular labyrinth

Facial nerve

Vestibular nerve

Auditory nerve

Oval window

Cochlea

With your head upright, the tiny embedded hairs are perpendicular in relation to the otoconia in your utricle.

If you tilt your head forward, the otoconia are pulled downward with the gel. The embedded hairs shift in the direction of the movement of the otoconia.

Mayo Clinic on Better Hearing and Balance   **209**

ear and musculoskeletal nerves are helping to keep you upright. However, in addition to having your eyes closed, if your central nervous system can't process the signals properly or if your vestibular labyrinth is not functioning, you may experience dizziness and possibly fall in the shower.

Causes of dizziness

Everyone has likely experienced brief episodes of dizziness at one point in his or her life. Momentary dizziness is often caused by an abrupt and rapid change in your environment.

Normally, your sense of balance is maintained subconsciously, based on years of practice and on healthy sensory input. For example, a toddler learning to walk is often quite unsteady and frequently loses his or her balance. But as the child gets older, the eye-muscle coordination becomes natural. Soon, walking and running doesn't require a second thought.

You may feel momentarily dizzy when your brain becomes aware of unusual sensory input, such as your first time on board a rocking boat. Another example is when you first get off a treadmill — it often takes a few seconds for you to adjust to the fact that your surroundings now move past you when you walk, in contrast to what happened during your workout.

Dizziness may also be the result of conflicting sensory information. For example, if you're sitting in a movie theater watching the shot of a landscape taken through the window of a speeding train, your eyes will be signaling movement. At the same time, your muscles, nerves and vestibular system indicate you're stationary. This can make you feel momentarily dizzy.

Spinning or sudden movements also cause feelings of dizziness. This happens because there's a brief lag when the fluid in your semicircular canals tries to catch up with the speed of your motion. When you stop moving, the fluid is still in motion, which makes you dizzy. When the fluid comes to rest, the dizziness generally goes away.

Dizziness caused by these changes generally isn't serious. But sudden, severe attacks or prolonged episodes of dizziness, faintness, lightheadedness or vertigo can be symptoms of an underlying disorder. Sometimes, it's the result of a disruption of your vestibular system. Other causes may include:

- **Low blood pressure.** Low blood pressure can make you feel light-headed or faint when you sit down or stand up too quickly (orthostatic hypotension).
- **Poor blood circulation.** Inadequate blood flow to the brain can make you feel lightheaded. Poor blood flow to the inner ear may cause vertigo. Poor circulation may be the result of a heart condition such as blocked arteries or irregular heartbeats (arrhythmia).
- **Multiple sensory deficits.** Lack of input from your eyes, nerves, muscles and joints can make you feel unsteady. Examples include failing vision, nerve damage in your arms and legs (peripheral neuropathy), osteoarthritis and muscle weakness.
- **Anxiety disorders.** These disorders include panic attacks and fear of leaving your home or being in large, open spaces (agoraphobia). They can make you feel spaced-out or lightheaded.
- **Hyperventilation.** Abnormally rapid breathing, which often accompanies anxiety disorders, can make you feel lightheaded.

- **Disorders of the central nervous system.** These include multiple sclerosis and tumors.
- **Migraines.** With or without head pain, migraine events are a common cause of dizziness.

Diagnostic tests

If you consult your doctor with a balance concern, you may be asked to undergo several tests that can assess the health of your inner ear and balance system. An audiologist usually performs these tests.

Test results can help determine if one or both ears are affected and how well your inner ear, eyes, muscles and joints work together. Your symptoms may also indicate whether you are a candidate for vestibular and balance rehabilitation therapy.

You'll likely be asked to not eat any food, consume alcohol and take any sedatives, tranquilizers or pain relievers for 24 hours before testing. You'll also want to wear comfortable clothing, such as pants or a sweat suit, as one of the tests (posturography) requires using a harness.

Should you be concerned about dizziness?

Generally, any unexplained recurrent or severe spell of dizziness warrants a visit to your doctor. Although it's uncommon for dizziness to signal a serious illness, see your doctor immediately if you experience dizziness or vertigo with any of the following:

- New, different or severe headache
- Blurred vision or double vision
- Hearing loss
- Speech impairment
- Leg or arm weakness
- Loss of consciousness
- Falling or difficulty with walking
- Numbness or tingling
- Chest pain or rapid or slow heart rate

These signs and symptoms may signal the development of a more serious problem, such as a brain tumor, stroke, Parkinson's disease, multiple sclerosis or heart disease.

Although the tests are simple and non-threatening, they're capable at times of making you feel dizzy, nauseated or anxious. Consult your audiologist with any concerns before, during or after testing. The examination may include one or more of the following tests:

Hearing test

Because the cochlea and vestibular labyrinth are both contained in the inner ear, problems with one structure often accompany problems with the other. The results of a hearing test may

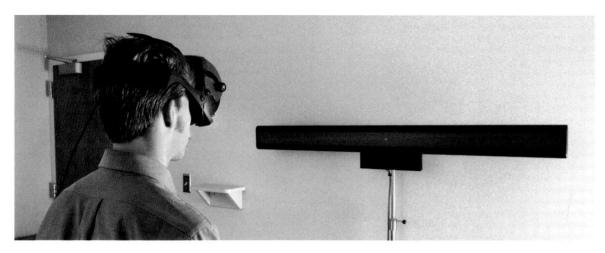

Videonystagmography

One part of videonystagmography involves following a pinpoint of light with your eyes as it moves across a horizontal electronic bar. This test evaluates how well the brain portions of your balance system control eye movements when your inner ear is not involved.

reveal something about your problems with balance. For a description of the standard hearing test, see Chapter 2.

Nystagmography

Nystagmography is actually a battery of tests that evaluates the interaction between your inner ear and your eye muscles — an interaction known as the vestibuloocular reflex.

Electronystagmography (ENG) is performed using electrodes to collect the information. Videonystagmography (VNG) uses tiny video cameras.

Whenever you turn your head, your inner ear signals the brain regarding this movement. The brain, in turn, signals your eye muscles in the vestibulo-ocular reflex. Essentially, your eyes will move in the opposite direction that you turn your head, permitting you to keep an object in a steady field of vision.

ENG and VNG detect nystagmus (nis-TAG-mus), or periods of uncontrolled, back-and-forth eye movements. Nystagmus may indicate a disorder or injury that's disrupting the vestibuloocular reflex. The tests are performed to study dizziness and vertigo.

For VNG tests, you may wear special goggles equipped with tiny infrared cameras that continually track the movement of your eyes. If the movements occur without any stimuli — for example, without you changing the position of your head — you may be experiencing nystagmus.

For ENG tests, instead of goggles, electrodes are taped at locations around your eyes to record the activity.

In order for the examiner to determine how well your eye movements will respond to signals from your inner ear, you may be asked to:

- Stare continuously at a fixed point of light or a spot
- Follow a point of light with your eyes as it moves back and forth along a horizontal bar
- Follow rotating points of light with your eyes
- Lie in different positions while your eye movements are recorded

Another test, known as the caloric test, involves warm water, cool water or air being circulated through a soft tube placed in your ear canal. The audiologist will observe your eye movements as different temperatures stimulate the inner ear.

Dix-Hallpike test

The Dix-Hallpike test can determine whether certain movements of your head trigger a form of vertigo known as benign paroxysmal positional vertigo (BPPV) — sudden, short bursts of vertigo (see page 218).

You'll start the test sitting on an examining table. The audiologist may study your eyes directly for the eye movements. Or you may be asked to wear special goggles equipped with cameras that display the eye movements on a video screen.

- The audiologist moves your head to the right or the left at an angle of about 45 degrees.
- You move quickly from a sitting position to lying down with your head extended over the edge of the table but still at the same angle and supported by the audiologist.
- The audiologist closely observes the movement of your eyes. If nystagmus occurs, it will indicate the location of the problem.

This procedure is done for both ears. If you have BPPV, you'll probably experience vertigo after two to 10 seconds of changing position. The sensation may last for 30 seconds to one minute. The direction of the nystagmus when you experience vertigo usually determines which ear is affected. The canalith repositioning procedure is usually successful in treating BPPV (see page 220).

Rotation tests

Rotation tests also detect your vestibuloocular reflex, but they tend to be more sensitive to inner ear problems. For example, they can monitor your control of eye movements while you're taking medications that may damage the inner ear (ototoxic medications) — which typically affect both ears. Not everyone will undergo rotation tests during a vestibular exam.

During testing, your audiologist may use electrodes or goggles equipped with infrared cameras to monitor your eye movements as your body is rotated in different directions and at various speeds. For safety, you're strapped into the chair with a harness and your head is secured against a headrest.

Typically, the testing room is darkened and your audiologist is seated at a computer console just outside the door. A microphone and headset allow you to maintain contact with the audiologist. Often, the computer-controlled

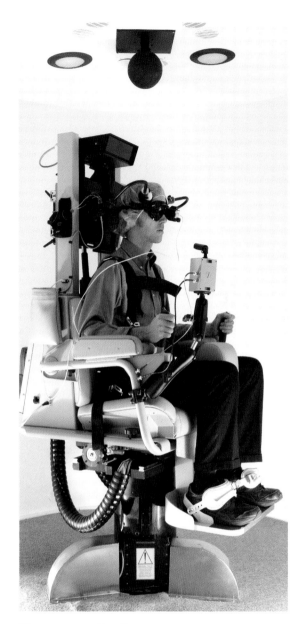

Rotary chair

During a rotation test, you'll sit in a rotary chair in a darkened room. The audiologist will monitor your eye movements while your body is rotated in the chair in different directions and at different speeds.

chair moves very slowly in a full circle. At faster speeds, it moves back and forth in a very small arc as your eye movements are recorded.

Rather than spinning the chair, the audiologist may have you focus on an object and voluntarily move your head from side to side or up and down for brief periods. Simplifying the test more, your audiologist may watch your eye movements while he or she manually moves your head or slowly spins you in a swivel chair.

Posturography

Posturography tests your ability to integrate the sensory information coming from different elements of your balance system: your eyes, the vestibular system in your inner ear, your muscles and joints, and the bottoms of your feet. The exam reveals which elements of the system you've come to rely on most for balance — either on their own or in combination with other elements.

To start the test, you'll be asked to remove your shoes and stand on a platform that detects changes in how you distribute your weight as you stand. This will help calculate the sway movements of your body to stay balanced.

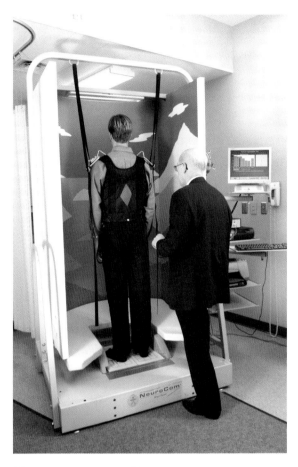

Posturography

This test measures how well you're able to maintain your balance in situations where your sensory systems have been slightly altered.

Wear comfortable clothes because you'll be slipping into a safety harness to make sure you don't fall. The audiologist will be standing close behind you in case you need some assistance to stabilize yourself.

During testing, varying conditions are created by altering one of your sensory systems. For example, you may be asked to remain balanced while your eyes are closed, or the platform you're standing on will no longer be stable and is set to rock with your body movements. The testing determines how well you're able to adjust to the changing circumstances.

Vestibular evoked myogenic potential

Vestibular evoked myogenic potential (VEMP) allows the audiologist to evaluate a specific part of the inner ear — the saccule, which is contained in the vestibular labyrinth (see page 209). Specifically, this test measures a neurological pathway between the inner ear and the brain known as the vestibulocollic reflex — a different reflex from the one studied in nystagmography.

You start the test seated. Several electrodes are taped to two large muscles in your neck. Earphones are worn that introduce loud clicking sounds to one ear or both ears. You'll be asked to press your head against a semi-inflated blood pressure cuff that's held in your hand. The pressure causes slight contractions in your neck muscles.

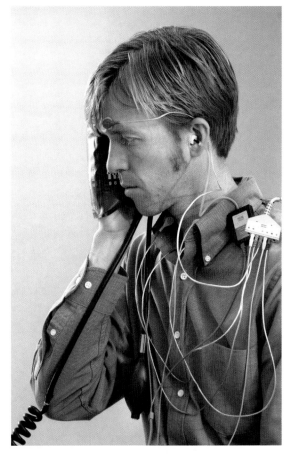

VEMP testing

For this test, you press a semifilled blood pressure cuff against your cheek to cause contractions of your neck muscles.

VEMP testing is useful for the detection of perilymph fistulas, particularly superior semicircular canal dehiscence (see pages 225-226). Research also suggests that VEMP testing may help diagnose Meniere's disease (see page 219).

Other tests

Magnetic resonance imaging (MRI) scans can reveal a variety of abnormalities — such as tumors — that may affect brain structures. Computerized tomography (CT) may be used to check for bone fractures or other skull abnormalities. Blood tests may be used to check for infection, and cardiovascular tests to check the health of your heart and blood vessels.

Vestibular disorders

Dizziness and, especially, vertigo — the sensation that your surroundings are whirling or spinning — are associated with vestibular disorders. The problem may arise from an infection in the inner ear or on the auditory nerve. It may also result from loose otoconia in the vestibular labyrinth (see page 209).

If you have a vestibular disorder, you may also experience nausea or vomiting, changes in heart rate and blood pressure, fear, anxiety and even panic. These effects may make you feel tired, depressed and lacking focus.

Most of the time, the vestibular problem is benign — which means it isn't life-threatening — and your doctor can prescribe ways to manage the condition. Some common vestibular disorders are described below:

Benign paroxysmal positional vertigo

Benign paroxysmal (buh-NINE par-ok-SIZ-mul) positional vertigo is commonly known by the abbreviation BPPV. This condition is a common cause of vertigo and more likely to occur in older adults.

BPPV is characterized by sudden, short bursts of vertigo — usually lasting less than a minute — that typically occur after you turn or change the position of your head. You may feel as if you're spinning or floating. Your eyes move back and forth involuntarily (nystagmus) while this happens. You may also experience nausea with rare occasions of vomiting, and lingering fatigue. Vertigo associated with BPPV may come and go unpredictably for weeks or even years.

Although the cause is unknown, BPPV is considered a mechanical problem of the balance system — and not a neurological problem with the sensory hair cells in the vestibular labyrinth or with the vestibular nerve. Sometimes a blow to the head precedes the condition, but BPPV may also occur spontaneously as a natural result of aging or from damage to the balance organ.

Regardless of the cause, scientists have learned that the tiny otoconia that are normally located in the utricle of the vestibular labyrinth break loose. Most often, these loose pieces accumulate in one of the semicircular canals.

Certain movements — such as rolling over in bed, sitting up or bending forward — move the particles, disturbing the fluid of the inner ear, which causes the hair cells in the canals to bend, setting off brief episodes of vertigo.

With the assistance of an audiologist, a simple procedure may be all it takes to manage BPPV. The canalith repositioning procedure involves maneuvers for positioning the head (shown on page 220). The goal is to progressively move the misplaced otoconia out of the canal to an open area near the utricle.

It may be necessary to repeat the procedure several times before the feeling of vertigo is eliminated. Afterward,

you'll need to keep your head upright for the rest of the day to help ensure that the particles stay out of the canal.

The canalith repositioning technique can be highly effective. However, a recurrence of vertigo frequently happens in the first year following a successful maneuver. If the symptoms do return, repeating the procedure usually helps. Therefore, it's important that individuals are instructed to perform the movements on their own to effectively manage the condition.

Meniere's disease

Meniere's (men-e-AYRZ) disease can affect adults at any age but is most likely to occur between 20 and 60 years of age. It's characterized by sudden attacks of vertigo, which may last anywhere from 20 minutes to several hours, but not longer than 24 hours.

The vertigo may make you feel nauseated or cause you to vomit. Other signs and symptoms of the condition include hearing loss, tinnitus and the feeling of a plugged ear. Vertigo is usually the worst symptom. You may be extremely sensitive to head movement, and the feeling of imbalance may continue from one to two days.

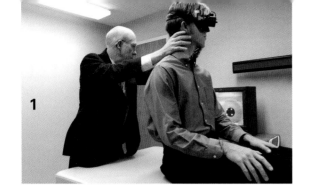

1

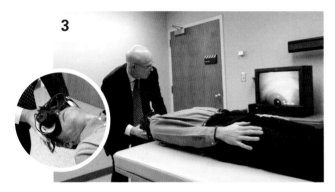

2

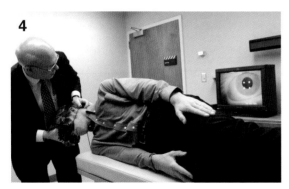

3

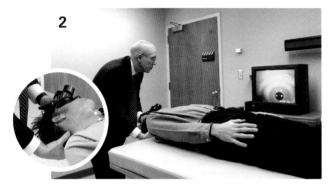

4

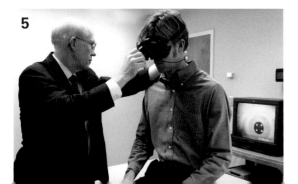

5

Canalith repositioning

To help relieve BPPV, your audiologist may help you perform a series of maneuvers. Each step is held for about 30 seconds. This example is for BPPV on your left side.

1. Start in a seated position with your head turned at a 45-degree angle to the left.
2. Move to a reclining position while your head is kept at the same angle. The audiologist supports your head as it extends over the edge of the table.
3. Still reclined, turn your head to the right.
4. Roll over on your side. Your head is angled slightly as you look down at the floor.
5. Return carefully to a sitting position with your chin tilted down.

Vestibular labyrinth

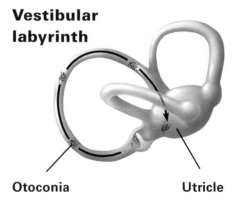

Otoconia   Utricle

As you work through procedure, the loose otoconia return to the area of the utricle.

Attacks may occur as frequently as every day or as infrequently as once a year. Between attacks, you usually feel back to normal. Although your ability to hear typically fluctuates with the attacks, the degree of hearing loss may gradually worsen. Meniere's disease usually affects only one ear, although it may affect both ears in about 25 percent to 30 percent of cases.

The cause of Meniere's disease is unknown, but scientists believe it's associated with fluctuations in the volume of fluid in the inner ear, as well as with the content of the fluid.

Treating Meniere's disease involves taking medications to manage the dizziness and nausea, and consuming a low-salt diet. Limiting your salt intake can help decrease the level of fluid in your body — and possibly the level in your inner ear — and decrease the frequency of attacks. Your doctor may also prescribe a diuretic to help you accomplish this.

If you experience frequent episodes of vertigo, your doctor may inject a small quantity of an antibiotic called gentamicin into your middle ear. Gentamicin is capable of causing inner ear damage, but in controlled amounts can reduce the activities of your vestibular system and control vertigo while leaving hearing intact. If dizziness is so severe that it inhibits your daily life, inner ear surgery may also be an option.

Labyrinthitis

Labyrinthitis is an inflammation of the inner ear — also known as the labyrinth — affecting both your balance and your hearing. The inflammation often follows the development of a bacterial ear infection or a viral upper respiratory illness. It may also occur after head trauma, or by itself with no other associated illness.

Signs and symptoms of labyrinthitis include sudden, intense vertigo that may last for several days, nausea and vomiting, nystagmus, hearing loss and tinnitus. If the inflammation is associated with a bacterial infection, you may experience a total loss of hearing in the affected ear.

Most of the time, the inflammation will go away on its own after a few weeks. Nevertheless, it's still important that you consult your doctor. To keep the symptoms of labyrinthitis from getting more severe, it's helpful during the initial days at the onset to remain as still

Surgery for vestibular disorders

Vertigo and other symptoms of vestibular disorders are most often treated with medications or through rehabilitation therapy, but surgery may also be an option. Which option is decided on will depend on the frequency and severity of your symptoms, the amount of hearing you've retained, your over-all health and your wishes. Some of the more common surgical procedures for vestibular disorders include:

- Patching a tear in either the oval window or the round window leading from the middle ear to the inner ear (perilymph fistula).
- Placing tissue over a tear at the top of one of the semicircular canals or blocking the canal (superior semicircular canal dehiscence).
- Draining excess fluid (endolymph) from the endolymphatic sac that's located near the mastoid bone behind your ear. This is called endolym-phatic decompression surgery.
- Cutting the vestibular nerve (vestibular nerve section) at a location before it joins with the auditory nerve. This procedure can potentially eliminate vertigo while preserving your hearing. It may be a reasonable option for a younger person with severe symptoms of Meniere's disease and no other significant medical problems.
- Destroying the inner ear (labyrinthectomy). This is a relatively simple oper-ation with fewer risks than in vestibular nerve section. Because the proce-dure involves destruction of the labyrinth, it's usually reserved for those who have no usable hearing in the affected ear. After surgery, the brain gradually adjusts, compensating for the loss of the balance mechanism in one ear by relying on the functioning mechanism of the other ear.

as possible and to avoid sudden changes in your position. This is also true for treating Meniere's disease during an attack of vertigo and for treating vestibular neuronitis.

If the problem underlying labyrinthitis is a bacterial one, the doctor will likely prescribe antibiotics to help get rid of the infection. Steroids may be given if there's no evidence of infection. If the condition is diagnosed within 72 hours of onset, the doctor may prescribe antiviral drugs.

Your doctor may also recommend medications to relieve dizziness and nausea. In some cases, a brief hospitalization is necessary due to the risk of dehydration from severe vomiting. Vestibular and balance rehabilitation will often help you manage symptoms associated with imbalance and head movement sensitivity.

Vestibular neuronitis

The symptoms of vestibular neuronitis are similar to labyrinthitis — both conditions cause a sudden onset of vertigo in addition to nausea, vomiting and nystagmus. Indeed, the two medical terms are sometimes — mistakenly — used interchangeably.

Both conditions may be caused by a viral infection, but whereas labyrinthitis is an infection of the inner ear, vestibular neuronitis is an infection of the vestibular nerve that connects the inner ear to the brain. Labyrinthitis may cause hearing loss, and vestibular neuronitis does not.

Signs and symptoms of vestibular neuronitis may last from several days to weeks, being severe at first and then gradually improving. Often, vestibular neuronitis will develop after a cold or other upper respiratory viral infection.

Most people recover completely from the neuronitis, although some may experience mild imbalance after the infection has been resolved.

Your doctor may prescribe medications to suppress the vertigo and nausea and steroids such as prednisone to help reduce inflammation. Your doctor may also prescribe vestibular and balance rehabilitation to help in your recovery (see pages 226-228).

Reactions to medications

The action of certain medications can damage the organs of hearing and balance in your inner ear. For this reason, these medications are considered oto-toxic (*oto* means "ear"). A list of common ototoxic drugs is in Chapter 5.

The effects of these medications, which can range from mild to severe, often depend on the doses you're taking and the length of time you take them, as well as factors such as your kidney and liver functions. Signs and symptoms of ototoxicity include:

- Onset of tinnitus in one or both ears
- Worsening of existing tinnitus
- A feeling that one or both ears are plugged
- Loss of hearing or worsening of existing hearing loss
- Blurred vision when you move your head
- Loss of balance

Make sure that your doctor is aware of any balance or hearing problem whenever you go for a medical visit. Report if you're experiencing balance problems after taking certain medications. This could help you avoid unnecessary exposure to ototoxic drugs.

Imbalance may persist following use of some medications. Vestibular and balance rehabilitation can teach you how to adjust to and cope with the ongoing loss of balance (see page 226).

The use of alcohol can cause vertigo and nystagmus, but these symptoms are temporary and will disappear once the alcohol's effects have subsided. However, the effect of alcohol can last up to 24 hours. Prolonged alcohol abuse can damage parts of your brain and result in permanent imbalance.

Acoustic neuroma

An acoustic neuroma, also known as a vestibular schwannoma, is a slow-growing, benign tumor that develops on what's known as the eighth cranial nerve — made up of the vestibular nerve and auditory nerve together.

The tumor develops as a result of over-production of certain cells, known as Schwann cells, that cover the nerves (see illustration on page 91). What causes the overproduction is unknown.

Hearing loss in one ear and tinnitus are common signs and symptoms of the disorder. As the tumor grows, it can affect other nerves that lead to your face, causing facial numbness and facial weakness. Although the vestibular nerve and blood supply to the balance organ are involved, the tumor grows slowly enough that imbalance and vertigo are rare symptoms.

Despite slow growth, it's possible for an acoustic neuroma to grow big enough to push up against the brainstem and interfere with life-sustaining functions. Your doctor may detect the acoustic neuroma with the use of magnetic resonance imaging (MRI). The tumor can be removed surgically or treated with radiation therapy.

Perilymph fistula

Perilymph fistula refers to the leakage of perilymph, a fluid from the inner ear, into the air-filled middle ear. The leakage occurs through a small tear in either the oval window or round window, which are thin membranes separating the middle ear and inner ear.

The condition most commonly results from trauma to the head, but may also be caused by rapid changes in atmospheric pressure — such as that experienced while scuba diving or doing airplane maneuvers. It may also occur due to extreme exertion — such as that needed for heavy lifting or childbirth.

The condition is controversial because the holes or defects in the membrane are so small and exceedingly difficult to detect — which can often call a diagnosis into question.

Signs and symptoms of perilymph fistula may include vertigo, imbalance, nausea and vomiting. A fistula may also lead to tinnitus and hearing loss.

Bed rest and avoiding sudden movements often allow the rupture to heal on its own. If this doesn't work, surgery may be performed to repair the tiny opening.

Superior semicircular canal dehiscence

Superior semicircular canal dehiscence (SSCD) is a type of perilymph fistula involving an abnormal opening in the inner ear. But with SSCD, the opening is at the top of one of the semicircular canals of the vestibular labyrinth, where there's a lack of bone covering the canal.

The primary symptom associated with SSCD is dizziness when straining — for example, when lifting something heavy — or when hearing loud noises such as dog barks. The condition may involve a specific type of hearing loss.

While not easy to diagnose, SSCD is far less controversial than an oval or round window fistula. That's because the opening on the semicircular canal can be detected with a CT scan or from certain audiological tests. Surgery can often repair the defect, relieving dizziness and returning your hearing to normal levels.

Vestibular rehabilitation

Dizziness and vertigo frequently go away on their own. But sometimes they persist. If you experience dizziness, vertigo or other signs and symptoms of a vestibular disorder that disrupt your life for several weeks or more, your doctor may refer you to a physical therapist for vestibular and balance rehabilitation.

This is an effective therapeutic program that uses physical exercise to decrease your symptoms and help you regain your sense of balance. Vestibular and balance rehabilitation is frequently recommended after inner ear surgery.

Compensation

The goals of this therapy are to stay active and to learn to maintain your everyday routine despite the balance concerns. This effort will help the normal mechanisms within your brain and central nervous system and your musculoskeletal system adapt to the changes you're experiencing. This adaptation is known as compensation.

When your vestibular system is damaged, your brain receives conflicting messages about movement and your body's position in space. That causes the dizziness or vertigo. You may try to avoid rapid movements at first in order to avoid these symptoms. But remaining relatively inactive for long periods of time doesn't stimulate your brain to change and adapt.

Adaptation often occurs naturally with experience, as you move around and carry out daily activities. In order for your brain to adapt, it needs to continue receiving signals from the balance organs — even if the signals are abnormal. Eventually, your brain resets itself to other sources of sensory input.

For example, if your inner ear on the left side stops functioning, your balance system may gradually switch to a heavier reliance on the organs of your right ear. When compensation is complete, you'll rarely notice the dizziness and vertigo anymore.

Anti-vertigo medications are important for relieving acute spells of dizziness, but long-term therapeutic use is discouraged. That's because these medications are mostly sedative in nature and may, in the long run, delay the ability of your brain to compensate.

At times the signs and symptoms of a balance disorder become chronic, which increases your risk of falling and injuring yourself. In older adults, falls are a major cause of disability and death. Thus, vestibular and balance rehabilitation can be an important factor in the prevention of falls.

What's in a program?

A vestibular and balance rehabilitation program generally starts with a thorough assessment of signs and symptoms and underlying conditions. This allows a physical therapist to design an exercise program customized to your needs. The assessment typically includes:

- Musculoskeletal evaluation to assess your strength, coordination and flexibility skills
- Balance and gait assessments that are compared with those of others in your age group and that test the interaction of your balance organs

- Questions about the frequency and severity of your symptoms, when and where they occur, and what factors might make them worse
- Rating your level of dizziness and vertigo as you change in and out of various positions
- Assessment of your ability to control eye movement while your head is in motion

With a better understanding of your situation, the therapist can help you set goals for the therapy, such as improving your eye movement control and increasing your activity levels. The therapist can also advise you on how to accomplish these goals.

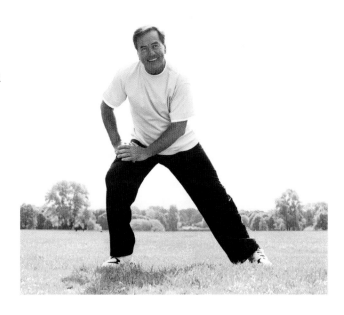

Typically, your therapist will recommend a number of exercises that you can do at home on a regular basis, in between visits to the physical therapy center. For example, you may be requested to do exercises in which you focus on a visual target 5 to 10 feet away while moving from a sitting position to a standing position and back again with your eyes open. You may then be asked to repeat the procedure with your eyes closed.

Other simple exercises may include watching a target at arm's length and moving your head quickly to the right and left while keeping the target in focus. This activity can be repeated several times a day.

At first, these exercises may make you dizzy, and you usually start out doing only a few repetitions at a time. Soon, your brain will become accustomed to the movements — it will find ways to compensate for your vestibular injury. You'll gradually increase the duration and intensity of the exercises. As you continue your program, the dizziness and vertigo will begin to fade away.

You also may be given exercises to increase your strength and coordination of muscle responses — to improve your balance control. This might include a daily walking program.

The best general suggestion is getting back to your normal, active daily routine as quickly as you can.

Staying active

Even after you finish a formal therapy program, it's important to stay physically active. If your body goes through a period of inactivity, such as during a bout with the flu or after minor surgery, your brain may forget some of its compensation methods.

To correct this, you'll need to retrain your balance system. This can be done by regularly performing the exercises that were initially prescribed to you, until the dizziness and vertigo go away. Generally, the signs and symptoms will recede more quickly the second time around.

For many individuals, tia chi has been helpful as a way of maintaining leg strength and balance after vestibular compensation is complete. It's often included as part of an active therapy program — but talk to your doctor before starting any exercise program.

Additional resources

Contact these organizations for more information about hearing loss, hearing aids, cochlear implants and problems with dizziness and imbalance. Some groups offer free publications or videos. Others have publications or videos you can purchase.

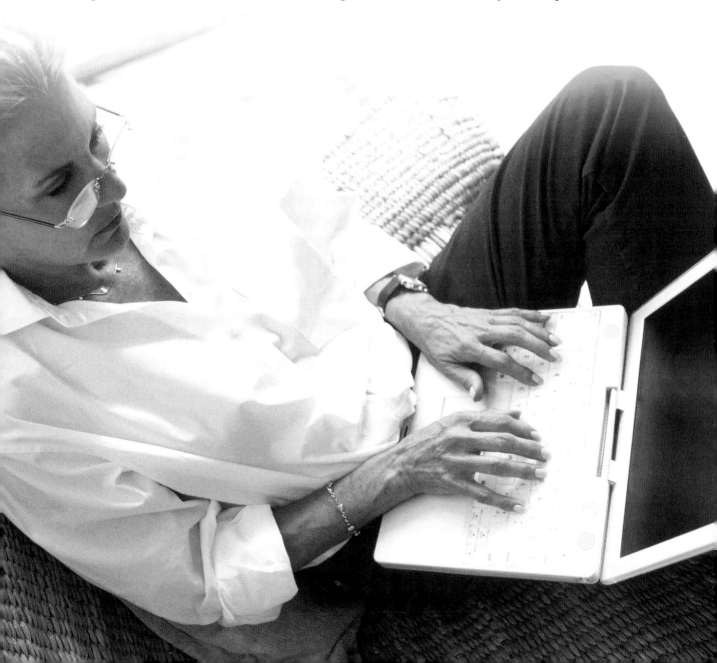

Alexander Graham Bell Association for the Deaf and Hard of Hearing
3417 Volta Place NW
Washington, DC 20007
(202) 337-5220 or (202) 337-5221 (TDD)
www.agbell.org

American Academy of Audiology
11730 Plaza America Drive, Suite 300
Reston, VA 20190
(703) 790-8466 or (800) 222-2336
www.audiology.org

American Academy of Otolaryngology — Head and Neck Surgery
1 Prince St.
Alexandria, VA 22314
(703) 836-4444
www.entnet.org

American Association of People with Disabilities
1629 K St. NW, Suite 503
Washington, DC 20006
(202) 457-0046 or (800) 840-8844
www.aapd-dc.org

American Auditory Society
352 Sundial Ridge Circle
Dammeron Valley, UT 84783
(435) 574-0062
www.amauditorysoc.org

American Hearing Research Foundation
8 S. Michigan Ave., Suite 814
Chicago, IL 60603-4539
(312) 726-9670
www.american-hearing.org

American Society for Deaf Children
3820 Hartzdale Drive
Camp Hill, PA 17011
(717) 703-0073 or (866) 895-4206
www.deafchildren.org

American Speech-Language-Hearing Association
2200 Research Blvd.
Rockville, MD 20850-3289
(800) 638-8255
www.asha.org

American Tinnitus Association
65 S.W. Yamhill St., Suite 200
Portland, OR 97207
(503) 248-9985 or (800) 634-8978
www.ata.org

Association of Late-Deafened Adults
8038 Macintosh Lane
Rockford, IL 61107
(815) 332-1515 or (866) 402-2532
www.alda.org

Better Hearing Institute
1444 I Street NW, Suite 700
Washington, DC 20005
(202) 449-1100
www.betterhearing.org

Canine Companions for
Independence
P.O. Box 446
Santa Rosa, CA 95402-0446
(866) 224-3647 or (800) 572-2275
www.caninecompanions.org

Children of Deaf Adults
Coda International
P.O. Box 30715
Santa Barbara, CA 93130-0715
www.coda-international.org

The Children's Hearing Institute
310 East 14th St.
New York, NY 10003
(212) 614-8380
www.childrenshearing.org

Dangerous Decibels
Oregon Health & Science University
3181 S.W. Sam Jackson Park Road
NRC04
Portland, OR 97201-3098
(503) 494-0670
www.dangerousdecibels.org

Deafness Research Foundation
641 Lexington Ave.
New York, NY 10022
(212) 328-9480 or (866) 454-3924
www.drf.org

Hearing Loss Association of America
7910 Woodmont Ave., Suite 1200
Bethesda, MD 20814
(301) 657-2248
www.shhh.org

International Hearing Society
16880 Middlebelt Rd., Suite 4
Livonia, MI 48154
(734) 522-7200
www.ihsinfo.org

League for the Hard of Hearing
50 Broadway, Sixth Floor
New York, NY 10004
(917) 305-7700 or (917) 305-7999 (TDD)
www.lhh.org

National Association of the Deaf
8630 Fenton St., Suite 820
Silver Spring, MD 20910-3819
(301) 587-1788 or (301) 587-1789 (TDD)
www.nad.org

National Center for Rehabilitative Auditory Research
3710 S.W. US Veterans Hospital Road
Portland, OR 97239
(503) 220-8262, Ext. 57991
www.ncrar.research.va.gov

National Institute on Deafness and Other Communication Disorders
National Institutes of Health
31 Center Drive, MSC 2320
Bethesda, MD 20892-2320
(800) 241-1044 or (800) 241-1055 (TDD)
www.nidcd.nih.gov

Paws With A Cause
4646 S. Division
Wayland, MI 49348
(616) 877-7297 or (800) 253-7297
www.pawswithacause.org

Vestibular Disorders Association
P.O. Box 13305
Portland, OR 97213-0305
(503) 229-7705 or (800) 837-8428
www.vestibular.org

Glossary

A

acoustic neuroma. Slow-growing, benign tumor on the auditory and vestibular nerves.

acoustic reflex. Muscle contraction in the middle ear that helps protect you from loud noise.

air conduction. How sound waves travel through the air-filled ear canal to reach the eardrum.

amplitude. Quality of sound, also known as loudness, that indicates the level of disturbance in a sound pressure wave. It's measured in decibels (dB).

assistive listening device (ALD). Device designed to help a person with hearing loss hear alerts and signals — such as telephones and alarm clocks — as well as converse in difficult listening environments.

assistive listening system. Technology that improves the sound quality and volume of pub-lic-address systems for people with hearing loss.

audiogram. Graph from an audiometric test that indicates your hearing thresholds for pure tones.

audiologist. Specialist trained to identify and measure hearing loss and vestibular disorders.

audiometry. Tests that measure your ability to hear pure tones and determine the faintest sounds you can hear.

auditory brainstem response (ABR). Measurement of electrical impulses sent from the inner ear to the auditory portions of the brain.

auditory cortex. Section of the brain, located in each temporal lobe, that processes electrical signals from the auditory nerve.

auditory nerve. Neurological pathway from the inner ear to the brain.

aural rehabilitation. Therapeutic program that helps you adjust to hearing loss.

autoimmune inner ear disease (AIED). Condition when your body's immune system attacks normal cells in your inner ear.

B

balance. Body system that allows you to know where you are in the environment and to maintain a desired position. It results from the interworking of your brain, inner ear, eyes, muscles and nerves.

barotrauma. Condition, also called airplane ear, resulting from unequal pressure between your middle ear and the outside environment.

basilar membrane. Structure in the cochlea that supports the organ of Corti and responds to the incoming sound waves.

behind-the-ear (BTE) hearing aid. Type of hearing aid with a circuitry casing that rests behind the ear.

benign paroxysmal positional vertigo (BPPV). Condition characterized by sudden, short bursts of vertigo.

binaural. Ability to hear sounds with both ears. This is important for good hearing and critical for locating the source of sounds.

biofeedback. Relaxation technique to help improve symptoms associated with many medical conditions.

Bone-anchored hearing aid (BAHA). Type of hearing aid attached to your skull that uses bone conduction to help you hear.

bone conduction. How sound waves travel through the bones of the skull to reach the inner ear.

C

caloric test. Test that observes eye movement as different water temperatures stimulate your inner ear.

canalith repositioning. Series of maneuvers undertaken to relieve symptoms of BPPV.

captioned telephone. Telephone equipped with a text screen that displays captions of real-time spoken conversation, used with a telecommunication relay service.

captioning. Display of spoken dialogue and sounds as printed words on a screen or monitor.

central auditory processing disorder. Malfunction in the auditory processing centers of your brain.

cerumen (earwax). Protective wax that forms in the ear canal.

cholesteatoma. Benign tumor found in the middle ear.

cochlea. Structure of the inner ear that translates sounds into electrical signals sent to the brain.

cochlear implant. Sophisticated technology that bypasses damaged parts of your inner ear by relaying electrical impulses directly to the auditory nerve. These impulses can be translated by the brain into sounds. The device is used by individuals with severe to profound hearing loss or no hearing.

cognitive behavioral therapy. Therapeutic program that attempts to help change your perceptions of a condition rather than the direct physical effects of the condition.

communications assistant (CA). Third-party operator in a telecommunications relay service who provides a bridge between the text and voice portions of a telephone conversation.

compensation. Your body's natural attempt to correct the malfunction or loss of an organ by increasing the functional capability of another organ or the unimpaired portions of the same organ.

completely-in-the-canal (CIC) hearing aid. Small hearing aid that fits inside the ear canal.

conductive hearing loss. The obstruction of sound waves due to blockage in the ear canal, ruptured eardrum or problems in the middle ear, resulting in hearing loss.

cued speech. Technique that supplements speech reading with the use of "cues" — specific hand shapes and placements around the mouth.

D

decibel (dB). Unit of measure that indicates sound intensity based on sound pressure level (dB SPL). Decibels also measure how a person's hearing compares with normal hearing (dB HL).

Dix-Hallpike test. Test to determine whether you have BPPV.

dizziness. Term to describe a variety of sensations associated with poor balance, including lightheadedness, unsteadiness and vertigo.

E

ear canal. The inch-long, air-filled pathway leading to the eardrum.

eardrum. Thin, taut membrane covering the entrance to your middle ear. Also called tympanic membrane.

earmold. Hearing aid earpiece that fits snugly into the ear canal.

ear, nose and throat (ENT) physician. Another name for an otolaryngologist or otologist.

electronystagmography (ENG). Battery of tests that evaluate the interaction between your inner ear and eye muscles.

eustachian tube. Narrow channel that connects the middle ear with the nose and throat.

F

feedback. High-pitched whistle or squeal that's made when an amplified sound is re-amplified.

FM system. Assistive listening technology that transmits sounds via radio waves to portable receivers worn by members of the audience.

frequency. Quality of sound, also known as pitch, that indicates how often a sound pressure wave fluctuates within a given amount of time. It's measured in hertz (Hz), or cycles per second.

frequency response. Range of frequencies to which a device such as a hearing aid can respond.

G

glomus jugulare tumor. Tumor that may grow in the middle ear and interfere with the ossicles.

H

hair cell. Cell in the cochlea that converts sound waves into electrical impulses carried to the brain. A hair cell in the vestibular labyrinth responds to motion.

hearing aid. Personal electronic device that amplifies sound.

hearing dog. Service dog trained to alert you to sounds such as telephones, doorbells and fire alarms.

hearing threshold. Faintest sound you can hear, usually measured across a range of frequencies.

hyperacusis. Extreme aversion to sound, including traffic noise, telephone rings and even normal conversations. The cause of this condition is unknown.

I

induction loop system. Assistive listening technology that transmits sounds via an electromagnetic field created by a loop of wire installed around the listening audience.

infrared system. Assistive listening technology that transmits sounds via light waves to portable receivers worn by members of the audience.

Internet protocol (IP) relay service. Internet-based telecommunications relay service that links telephones and computers.

in-the-canal (ITC) hearing aid. Type of hearing aid that fits partly in the ear canal but extends to the bowl of the outer ear.

in-the-ear (ITE) hearing aid. Type of hearing aid that fills most of the bowl of your outer ear.

L

labyrinthitis. Inflammation of the inner ear, which can affect the cochlea and vestibular labyrinth.

M

masker. Device that adds subtle background noise in order to help cover over, or mask, tinnitus.

mastoid bone. Projection of bone in the skull that lies behind the ear.

mastoidectomy. Surgical removal of diseased mastoid bone.

Meniere's disease. Disease characterized by attacks of vertigo, hearing loss and tinnitus.

middle ear. Air-filled cavity between the eardrum and inner ear that contains the ossicles.

mixed hearing loss. Combination of both sensorineural and conductive hearing loss.

myringotomy. Procedure in which a small incision is made in your eardrum to equalize pressure and remove fluid from your middle ear.

N

nasopharynx. Upper part of the throat linked to the ear by the eustachian tube.

nystagmus. Involuntary back-and-forth movement of the eyes, which may indicate a vestibular disorder.

O

open-fit-behind-the-ear hearing aid. Smaller version of the behind-the-ear hearing aid that leaves the ear canal partially open — allowing you to use the remaining good hearing in that ear.

organ of Corti. Structure in the cochlea with hair cells that convert sound to electrical impulses.

ossicles. Three tiny bones (hammer, anvil and stirrup) in the middle ear that transfer sound to the inner ear.

ossicular chain disruption. Displacement or fracture of the ossicles, often due to trauma.

otitis media. Middle ear infection that occurs when the eustachian tube becomes blocked and fluid that builds up becomes infected.

otoacoustic emission (OAE). Inaudible but measurable sounds created in the cochleas of people with normal hearing — but not in people with hearing loss.

otoconia. Tiny particles in the vestibular labyrinth that respond to the acceleration of movements, stimulating the hair cells.

otolaryngologist. Doctor trained to diagnose diseases of the ear, sinuses, mouth, throat, and other structures of the head and neck.

otologist. Otolaryngologist who has specialized in ear disorders.

otosclerosis. Condition in which a growth of spongy bone immobilizes the stirrup, causing conductive hearing loss.

otoscopy. Examination of the ear canal, eardrum and middle ear that's performed with an otoscope equipped with a light.

ototoxic. Term indicating something that's harmful to your hearing.

oval window. Membrane separating the inner ear from the middle ear, in addition to the round window.

P

perforation. Hole or tear in the eardrum, often accompanied by pain, bleeding or discharge.

perilymph fistula. Leakage of fluid from the inner ear to the middle ear, sometimes a result of head trauma.

pinna. Cupped section of the outer ear that gathers sound waves from your surrounding environment.

posturography. Test to assess your balance when one or more of your senses is blocked.

presbycusis. Hearing loss associated with aging that develops when hair cells within your cochlea wear out.

R

reverberation. Echo effect produced when sound waves are reflected multiple times off hard surfaces, causing the sound to persist. A primary cause of hearing problems in public spaces.

rotation test. Test that monitors eye movements in relation to your body rotation.

round window. Membrane separating the inner ear from the middle ear, in addition to the oval window.

S

saccule. Chamber in the vestibular labyrinth that helps monitor the vertical movements of your head in relation to the ground.

semicircular canal. Any of three tubes that form the vestibular labyrinth. The fluid-filled canals contain hair cells that assist your sense of balance.

sensorineural hearing loss. Hearing loss, often permanent, that results from damage to the inner ear or the auditory nerve.

sign language. Complete language of hand signs, body movements, gestures, facial expressions and other visual cues to form words.

speech processor. Computer chip in a cochlear implant that converts sounds from the environment into coded electronic impulses.

speech reading. Technique, also known as lip reading, for recognizing spoken words by watching movements of the speaker's lips, tongue, jaw, eyes and eyebrows.

speech reception threshold (SRT). Faintest level at which you can understand spoken words at least half the time.

speech spectrum. Concave depiction on an audiogram that represents the sounds that make up human speech.

stapedotomy. Surgery to treat otosclerosis with a prosthesis.

sudden sensorineural hearing loss (SSNHL). Severe hearing loss in the inner ear that occurs all at once or within a few days.

superior semicircular canal dehiscence (SSCD). Form of perilymph fistula involving the loss of bone covering the superior semicircular canal.

swimmer's ear. Infection of the ear canal, often due to moisture.

T

telecoil. Small circuit in a hearing aid that converts electromagnetic waves into sound, allowing you to hear clearly on the telephone.

telecommunications relay service (TRS). Public service that provides real-time communication on the telephone for individuals with hearing loss.

telecommunications device for the deaf (TDD). Telephone equipped with a display screen for the text of spoken words. The device is used by individuals with profound hearing loss or no hearing, with the assistance of a telecommunications relay service.

text messaging. Use of a phone keypad as a keyboard to send short messages to one or more other phones — also known as short messaging service (SMS).

timbre. Subjective quality of sound that allows you to distinguish between sounds of the same frequency and amplitude.

tinnitus. Perception of sound, such as a ringing or buzzing, in your ears. The condition can be objective (the sounds can be heard by others) or subjective (the sounds are heard only by the individual).

tinnitus retraining therapy (TRT). Therapeutic program that helps you become more accustomed to tinnitus so that the sound blends into the background.

tuning fork. Device that sounds a single tone and is helpful for assessing hearing loss.

tympanometry. Test to check function of the eardrum and middle ear.

U

utricle. Chamber in the vestibular labyrinth that helps monitor the horizontal movements of your head in relation to the ground.

V

ventilation tube. Small tube inserted into the eardrum to relieve ear pressure or a middle ear infection.

vertigo. Intense feeling that you or your surroundings are spinning or whirling.

vestibular and balance rehabilitation. Therapeutic program that uses exercise to help you regain your sense of balance.

vestibular evoked myogenic potential (VEMP). Test to assess the neurological pathway between the vestibular system and brain.

vestibular labyrinth. Structure of the inner ear that assists with your balance.

vestibular neuronitis. Inflammation of the vestibular nerve, producing symptoms similar to labyrinthitis.

W

word recognition testing. Test that determines how well you're able to understand single-syllable words at a comfortable volume.

A